Deadly Snakebite

A.C. Johnson

Deadly Snakebite
by A.C. Johnson

All Scriptures are taken from the New International Version, New Living Translation, and King James Version of the Bible, unless otherwise specified.

Author A.C. Johnson can be reached via email at johnops51@yahoo.com

CONTENTS

Introduction

Introduction

There are two creations of God which mankind cannot afford to ignore, for both provide a fata fascination to mankind. Mankind [male-kind] may like them, or fear them, but can never overlook or ignore them. These two creations have some things in common. They use their tongues a lot, change their wardrobes often, and change the directions of their destination and direction suddenly.

They both undulate, and will not move forward in a straight line. It is not always safe to follow, or chase them, for they can let you catch up with them. It is then, that it becomes very dangerous to handle them unwisely. Many have lost their lives, and even more.

These two creations have influenced the entire human culture, the fashions of the world, and even the events of the world. History is full of their exploits, and their profound influence on mankind. We will talk about one of them in this presentation, the serpents, also called as snakes.

My introduction to snakes began when I was about 6 years old when I saw an unconscious man carried to be treated by a shaman called 'snake-bite healer' who lived across the house where I lived in India. I remember a lot of 'Mantras' [magic slogans] being shouted, followed later by wailing, and I suppose that the patient became a statistical number of snakebite victims.

Later as a young boy growing up, I came across numerous venomous and, non-venomous snakes especially during the summer holidays I spent in the foothills and forest edge, visiting my grandfather's home in the Kambam Valley.

– **A.C. Johnson**

Chapter 1

The Collegiate Bushman's Story

My physical birth took place in the year 1930, in Thanjavur, India. In the year 1946, I was born-again in my spirit in Tambaram, while I was doing my Intermediate college studies. This happened when I was met by a fleet-footed fellow student called Philip Asirvatham, who challenged me for a short run during which he beat me hollow. Later, he challenged me gently on my spiritual walk, or run, my understanding, and even my 'standing.' He said that he had become a believer in the true God, who can communicate with us personally, on an individual basis,

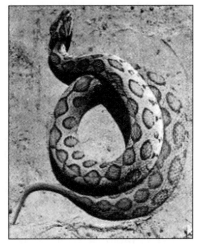

one on one. Happily for me, I lost in combating this challenge also, and ended up becoming a member of the seven 'bush-men' club, as my friend and his partners were called.

There were vast bush lands in the outskirts of the college campus, [Madras Christian College Tambaram] where Philip Asirvatham, Jobdas Daniel, George Rajaratnam, Thomas Paranjothi Ambrose, Whitson Paul, Joshua Daniel and I met every evening for prayer and meditation. The rest of the college students called this group as 'Bush-men of Tambaram'. Often the group returned to the hostel well after sunset. There is no twilight in that part of the world, and it gets very dark soon after sunset.

Many of us, including me walked bare footed, except when going to the college for attending classes. We ran, played basketball, field hockey, football etc bare footed. One evening while coming back from prayers, walking in real darkness without a flashlight, [flashlights were scarce in those days] I stepped on something that felt like a thick rope that rolled under my foot.

After reaching the hostel, I had the opportunity to talk to my neighbor about God's love and power. I had my feet up on a table, and my friend exclaimed in alarm that there were two puncture wounds in the sole of my foot, from which blood was seeping out. He thought that the punctured wounds looked like snakebite, and I remembered that I stepped on some thing ropy, a few minutes earlier.

My neighbor wanted to take me to the emergency room hoping to get some one to help. I declined, for strangely I was not alarmed and I told him that the doctor, who came to the emergency room, came only during the daytime, and that too only on certain days.

Even if I had sought medical help it would have been almost impossible to treat me as I did not see whether it was a viper, or an elapid like cobra that had probably bit me. All I could make out was that the puncture marks suggested a venomous snake rather than a non-venomous one. My neighbor kept a close watch on me for the rest of the evening to late night. He became receptive to our talks about spiritual matters, from then on.

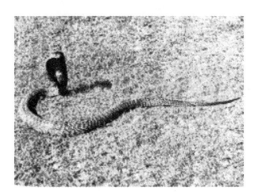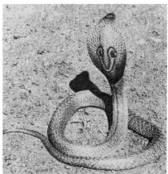

[Images Above: Cobras. Venom predominantly neuro-toxic. Paralyses respiratory muscles.]

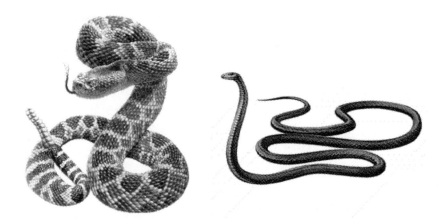

Rattlesnake, predominantly hemo-toxic venom (Left). Mamba, predominantly neuro-toxic venom (Right)

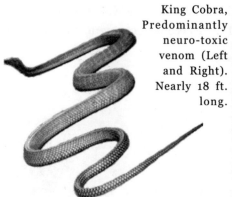

King Cobra, Predominantly neuro-toxic venom (Left and Right). Nearly 18 ft. long.

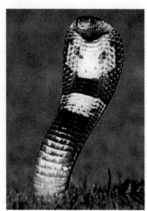

Chapter 2

Medical School and Herpetology

My next close encounter was when I was a medical student in the Christian Medical College in Vellore. I saw a big, thick snake out side the classroom, in the Medical College campus, and presumed it was a python because of its size. I hit it with a stick and thought that I had killed it. Our histology professor wanted to mount the head of the snake in a big glass jar. I offered to hold the neck of the snake while the lady professor [Dr. Holt] was cutting it below the neck.

The snake was only stunned, and came alive during the procedure. The mouth opened and large fangs came out, dripping venom. It was a powerful snake and trying to get free of my hand and would have killed us if I had not held on for dear life-literally. I found out later that it was the powerful dreaded Russell's viper.

The college campus was built at the foot of small hills of the Eastern Ghats [range of hills] of south Indian peninsula. I had a few

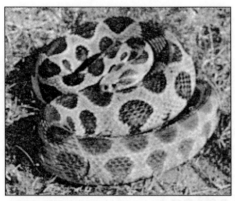

Russell's viper. Venom is predominantly hemo-toxic, tissues dissolve.

more encounters with poisonous snakes and I killed them, without being bitten.

My fascination for snakes was not confined to the physical snakes ranging over 2000 species, out of which only 10% were venomous, but more so to the 'spiritual' species, where all 100% are venomous. The physical snakes have venoms that are grouped into the following:

Neurotoxins disable a chemical called acetyle-choline, which helps nerve conduction between the nerve endings and in the muscles. This results in paralysis of the muscles, especially of the muscles involved in respiration [breathing]. The snake bitten person may need tracheotomy and ventilator support to help breathing. The toxins also affect the brainstem and the higher centers keeping a person alive while paralyzing them.

Hemotoxins contain a group of enzymes and proteins that affect the normal bleeding and clotting mechanisms. This results in protracted bleeding into various parts of the body.

Cardio toxins and cyto toxins adversely impair the cardiac muscles and the blood cells. This will cause cardiac arrest.

Myo-toxins and tissue-toxins contain proteins and enzymes that digest and cause muscle necrosis, and tissue necrosis. Even when the human victim is alive, he/she will experience necrosis and destruction within the body, and suffer the effects of bleeding into the stomach, intestines, and kidneys to mention a few.

The spiritual serpents have more potent venom. Humanity has developed antivenin against the various physically venomous snakes, which are moderately successful when administered in time. But humanity has not been able to find any antidote for the spiritual serpent venom. The only effective antidote will be discussed later in this book.

The spiritual serpent venom contains many toxins and only a few of these are listed below. Anger, is potent venom that contains many subgroups of venom in it. This venom was responsible for the first murder between brothers and cause for well over 90% of wars, murders, violence and bloodshed, from then to this date.

Pride is a fatal venom that also contains many subgroups of venoms under it.

Selfishness and self-centeredness are like venoms that destroy tissue.

Covetousness of various kinds are fatal venoms.

Sexual impurities of various types kill people in the prime of their lives.

The high level of casualty is because of denial, procrastination of treatment, or mislaid trust in the strength of the victim's own immune system, or invincibility. This has led to disregarding and rejecting God's offer to help and cure. This unfortunately is the most common cause of fatality.

Recommended and 'Not' recommended Treatments for Terrestrial Snakebites:

1.   Snake stones. There is a large market in many countries for cure for any venomous snakebite. Unfortunately for the believers, there is no proven cure by snake stones.

2. Pouring alcohol on the bite site, and pouring a larger amount into mouth has been tried. It has resulted in the victim being dead-drunk!

3. Herbs for snake bite. So far there is no proved herbal cure. The Irrullas, the snake catchers of India have some herbal combinations that seem to work, but it has been kept a secret so far.

4. Making a crucial cut at the snake bite site to let out the poison. This is not recommended in this day and age. A viper bite has venom that will make this incision a major bleeding site. The tissue necrosis will be aggravated by local infection.

5. Sucking the puncture and spitting out the venom does not work, and is dangerous for one with abrasions in the mouth of the sucker. Mechanical suction is acceptable.

6. Local cooling or cauterizing with heat or acid is not recommended, because of local tissue necrosis danger.

7. Applying a firm and not tight bandage or tourniquet 3-4 inches above the site is recommended to slow down venom spread. Possible only if the bite is on the extremity like arm or leg. One should be able to slip a finger between the tourniquet and the limb to allow for circulation.

8. The person should not run or walk, but if possible be taken on a stretcher quickly to the hospital. The victim should be encouraged to stay calm and covered up to minimize shock reaction. The part of bite should be kept well below the level of the heart.

9. All the above are only supplementary. The one and only effective and proved treatment is to give specific antivenin intravenously, taking precaution for allergic reaction.

In many countries, antivenin is prepared by using the venoms of mixture of different species of snakes [of Cobra, Russell's viper, Saw tooth viper and Krait], as many cannot identify the snake that bit them. In addition some of the snakes may carry the venom of a different species.

The spiritual serpent venom carries long-term fatality and is more prevalent as 100% of humanity has been bitten and envenomed. If you and I find any of the symptoms, we need to take immediate action. The choice of ignoring the bite, or patching it up to cover the bite or using stone or magic slogan techniques which are worthless, or, go to the one who offers. The real well proven antivenin treatment is yours? [We will deal with this later].

Chapter 3

Bulimic Balu

After graduating from the medical school, I came across a man performing with snakes on the roadside. He had a number of cobras, which were the usual part of his roadside snake show. The snake charmer usually blows on a home made pipe producing high-pitched weird sounds, referred to as snake music. During this time the cobras rear up with their hoods spread out and weave side to side, or back and forth, hypnotized by the rhythmic move ments of the pipe and the charmer's knee.

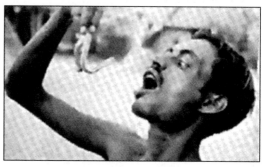

Balu ready to swallow
[a snaky snack!]

This performer was different, for he did not have the musical accompaniment; the significant second part of the show was when he swallowed 15 live water-snakes, each measuring two to three feet in

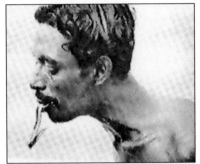

Balu regurgitating out one of the snake that was swallowed.

length, and 10 live frogs. After a short talk to his audience, he expelled the still alive snakes, and the frogs, one at a time, or in a bunch at a time. He carefully caught and bottled them up for the next show.

The man was a small skinny person. I thought that he was doing a mass hypnotic show. I took a few photos, as I was carrying my camera with me. I did my own film developing and printing, and made the enlargement of photos I liked. As soon as I went home, I processed the film and to my surprise, the enlarged prints showed that the snakes were coming out of the mouth of the man 'for real'!

I could hardly sleep that night. I had been working on the gastro-esophageal motility and in particular the gastro-esophageal reflux, called as GERD these days. I realized that this roadside performer has some thing to offer to the high academic medical knowledge, which was floundering in this area.

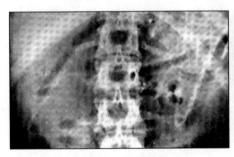

Snakes and frogs swimming in Balu's stomach

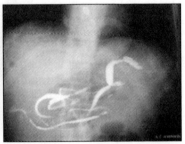

Live Snakes in Balu's Stomach outlined by barium fed to the snakes

Next morning I sent for Balu, the performer. I was in charge of the department of diagnostic Radiology at the Christian Medical

College Hospital at that time. We had a 35 mm Arryflex camera attached to the fluoroscopy- television module on a powerful X-ray machine.

I persuaded the nervous Balu, the roadside performer/teacher to get behind the Fluoroscopy unit and made him swallow the snakes and the frogs. Due to the rapid movements of the snakes and the frogs inside Balu's stomach, the details were poor when I did fluoroscope and took a plain x-ray of the abdomen of Balu.

Anticipating this, I had prepared Barium solution that is always given to the patients during the Upper Gastro-intestinal studies.

So I had the privilege of giving barium solution as Barium-meal to the non-poisonous water snakes, using a tube attached to a syringe containing Barium. I then asked Balu to give me his repeat show while I had him behind the fluoroscopy screen of the x-ray machine. I documented the findings on the 35 mm cine film using the Arryflex camera attached to the unit.

Chapter 4

Hiatus -
Hernia

Your stomach can jump-up, nearly to your mouth!

I had the Arriflex 35 mm camera attached to the fluoroscopy unit in order to do gastro-intestinal motility studies, various angiographic studies, and contrast studies of various organs. As mentioned earlier, at that time, I was doing a research on hiatus hernia and gastro-esophageal reflux. It was also the time when hiatus hernia surgical repair was extremely popular, done as the 'bread and butter' procedure, [after routine appendectomy and tonsillectomy became unpopular].

It was the time when the medical science considered

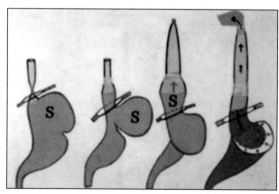

Diagrammatic picture of hiatus hernia and gastro-esophageal reflux

that hiatus hernia and gastro-esophageal reflux should be uncommon, dangerous, and or abnormal and needed surgical correction. I worked out a protocol for diagnosis of hiatus hernia, and found that the gastro-esophageal junction migrated up and down the hole called the 'hiatus' in the diaphragm very frequently [meaning that hiatus hernia is very common].

I found that gastro-esophageal reflux was also common, and the treatment for these two conditions is called for, only when complications set in. I was able to provide the parameters for surgery through an extensive research on many hundreds of patients coming for treatment to this caring, concerned hospital.

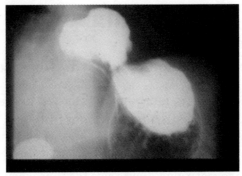

Voluntary production of a large size hiatus hernia,
reduced completely, voluntarily

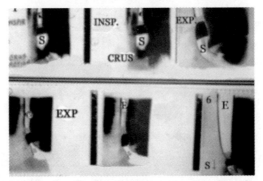

Crus is the diaphragm's purse-string that closes
around the esophago-gastric junction.

The crus closes during inspiration and opens during expiration. The above image shows an apprehensive patient with a small hiatus hernia showing effects of "Straining" and "Relaxing." The stomach returns to the abdomen during relaxation.

These findings of mine challenged the criteria for the then currently held medical and surgical opinions. I believe that Balu's performance was 'divinely' offered to the multitude of potential patients and to me, on a plate. The importance was increased as the esophageal symptoms overlapped symptoms related to serious heart disease, even serious heart attacks.

Even lung disorders such as asthma, and cough are evoked or precipitated by gastro esophageal reflux. For, the major parasympathetic nerves supplying the esophagus, stomach, part of the intestines, the lungs and the heart are part of a large nerve called the vagus nerve. Not only patients, but also physicians are often confused by these 'vague' symptoms of the 'vagus.'

Many tests are needed to differentiate the under lying problem. For, there is a merging and triggering of problems of one body system to another under vagus innervations. I had x-ray markers put in the junction of the esophagus and the stomach, and showed that the junction showed movement up into the chest when the patient became apprehensive, such as in a pre-surgical time and returned to normal position in the abdominal cavity post operatively. These were shown in patients who were not being operated to repair a hiatus hernia. I have documented these on still and movie studies.

Chapter 5

Gastro-Esophageal Reflux

You can spit from your stomach.

I had since then, found many other such roadside and circus performers who could "spit" from the stomach and studied them. I found that any one could regurgitate, or 'spit' from the stomach and can produce, and reduce a sizable hiatus hernia, at will, by simple practices.

My findings and report interested the surgeons, gastro-enterologists and radiologists around the world, and I was invited to speak, present, and defend my findings in many national and international meetings around the world.

The recurrent reflux of the gastric acid back into the esophagus, which is intended for transporting food mixed with the alkaline saliva from the mouth to the stomach, contained a high degree of acid. The esophagus, which has a normal squamus epithelial, lining, tends to get inflamed by the frequent acid baths. The inflammation can resolve

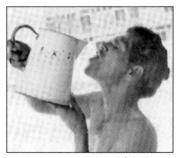
Appa Rao pours a jug of water into
his Stomach

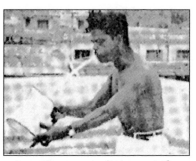
Appa Rao regurgitates out the
water back into the jug

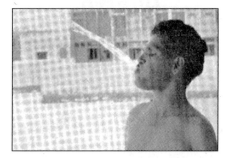
Appa Rao spouts the water like a fountain
from his stomach

or proceed to ulcer formations and scarring, causing strictures that need major surgical correction.

The other potential danger is when the esophageal mucosal lining starts to change and develop columnar mucosal lining as is present in the stomach. This action is called 'metaplasia,' which can precede an 'anaplasia,' a malignant change to develop into cancer. As the acid bathes the esophagus, the acid sensation causes a reflex action producing contraction of the longitudinal muscles of the esophagus, pulling the stomach into the chest cavity.

The stomach is normally located in the abdominal cavity. The above mentioned are the reasons for the hiatus herniation and gastro-

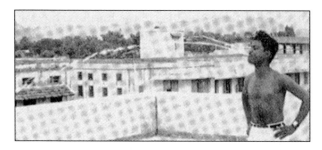

Appa Rao spouts the contents of the stomach full of water
to 10 feet plus distance

esophageal reflux. There are many aggressive approaches for patients with gastro-esophageal reflux and hiatus hernia.

But as I mentioned earlier, I found that even apprehension was enough to pull the gastro-esophageal junction into the chest cavity due to the wide spread action of the vagus nerve.

Many different kinds of repairs of the hiatus hernia have ended in a breakdown and recurrences of the hernia were observed and documented by my study as well as many others. By God's grace, these contributions did change the way of the treatment eventually, which was to the ultimate advantage of the patients, and to their wallets.

Balu was like the human 'Pavlov's Pouch' to study the physiology of secretions and motility of the upper gastro-intestinal system. I offered him a job in the department of Radiology, with a stable income and benefits, while I studied him. He stayed on with me for a few days, but became restless to be on the road to 'eke-out' meager pennies a day to satisfy his desire for 'freedom.'

As a young boy, he had run away from home with a visiting circus troupe, and loved a wandering nomadic type of life. I arranged many shows for him to keep him around while I was getting more clinical data.

Balu insisted on bringing his cobras into his shows every time. He would even bring the 'snake baskets' to keep in my office to take to the 'after work shows.' The lids of the baskets were flimsy, with no means of securing to keep them shut. The snakes could easily push the lid open!

I have seen Balu being bitten by the cobras a few times, and tried to get antivenin for him. But he refused, saying that he had the right antidote at home that he usually takes a small portion in the mornings, and if bitten, he would take the second dose of the oral antidote, which he kept 'safely' in his house. He would not tell me what the antidote was, though I offered him money to make it available for others. He said "one of these days, he would."

[But, sadly, as we all experience, the "one of these days" usually escapes us]. We need to do what we need to, this very day. Procrastination adversely influences our destination.

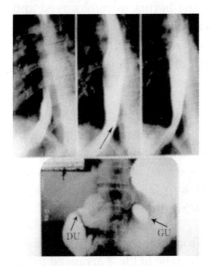

GASTRO-ESOPHAGIAL REFLUX & GASTRIC+DUODENAL ULCERS

I had to gather the money for his shows and give it to him, and added to the collection, when they were too small. Many times I told him that I and others around are at grave risk, as we do not have easy recourse to cobra bite. He said that the snakes he brings too close to me would be defanged.

I knew he only said that to soothe me down, and was not true. I had to tell him that the extracted main poison fangs do grow back, and if the venom glands are not removed, even the other teeth of the snake are enough to get the venom into a bite, to make it fatal.

I had to brush up on my science of 'herpetology' [study of snakes]. I tried to keep some antivenin handy, [1-2 vials] and tried to have a friend nearby to treat me if necessary. I realized that this was more a token than the necessary dosage. But it was not always possible to carry out even these precautions. I was aware that unless I had the specific antivenin for the type of snakebite, and that too in sufficient quantity, the risk was very high. But I was young, and my blood was hot, and taking risks was a heady wine I relished.

I got to know many great herpetologists including Dr. Wad, from Haffkine [snake] institute, Bombay, Mr. Rom Whitaker, now the founder of the crocodile and snake-park in Chennai, India, [featured by the National Geographic catching king cobras]; and Prof. Rajendran, an eminent zoologist, whose entire family members were herpetologists. His children had non-venomous snakes of many types in their house, while the Professor had the venomous types of many kinds in an 'out-house.'

The 'college going' daughters of the professor carried beautiful non-poisonous snakes in their handbags. I often wondered if the common pickpockets, burglars, and bag snatchers of India had an opportunity of robbing the family of the professor, and wished I was around at that time with my camera. I had a 16mm movie camera, and documented most of my studies as well as many venom-milking procedures, of different kinds of venomous snakes.

I was taking risks with close up shots. [I did make a documentary movie titled 'snakes in the service of mankind'] which is resting in a box since 1970, waiting till I get back my enthusiasm that got quenched after what happened to Balu.

The Bible says that one who keeps and uses the sword [for example, a soldier] will die by a sword.

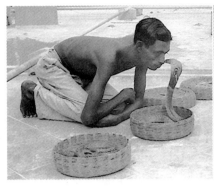
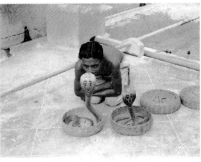

Balu and the Kiss of Death

It is a common knowledge that most of the snake handlers will be bitten by snakes, and only a few of those bitten by very venomous snakes live to tell the pain, agony and horror of experiencing the passage of the venom through their bodies, even when they were being treated under the best of medical facilities. [More on this matter, later.]

I understood that Balu must have developed significant immunity to cobra venom. I had real concerns whether giving him antivenin may produce a fatal 'anaphylactic reaction' in him, while he was under my care, and needed the antivenin treatment.

One day, I had a call from a friend, that Balu has been admitted into a hospital for snakebite. I was in Vellore, a town about 80 miles away. I called up the doctor attending on Balu and offered to pay for his treatment, and to take all efforts to save his life. But it was too late.

Later I heard that prior to this incident, Balu had got married, and had also hired a man to carry the snake baskets. Between that new assistant and the new wife, the 'two' removed, or, misplaced the antidote he usually took when bitten by the snake. Either-way, Balu could not find the antidote, and might have panicked and gone into a panic and shock. Or, more likely, the venom of the cobra that bit him had a different composition of venom against which he had no defense.

It was not only a loss to science, but also for me, as Balu had become a good friend by that time.

My work on this area became no more a pleasure and so I put them off on 'hold', because I had depended on human beings including my 'self' for my studies and research, and had not leaned on God who is really the 'author, and finisher' of all things. The fame or name that my work got for me, brought me under the spiritual serpent bite, and I was envenomed.

You may later hear about the signs and symptoms. It is vital that we get the right treatment through obtaining the antivenin prepared at the Cross without any delay.

Chapter 6

Serpent
in
the
Sky

The most ancient but the most up-to-date book of books, which has stood the test of time and remained the best seller and sought after, centuries after centuries, and has needed no updating and has offered a guideline for every aspect of human life, the Bible, [recognized as the Word of God] mentions Satan the spiritual serpent and, him biting humanity.

The Bible does not give us details about the rebellion and fall of Satan, an archangel, called as Lucifer a cherubim and music minister along with some of the angels.

We do not know when it happened or exactly why. [We presume it was even prior to the creation of the world.] Is it permissible for us to wonder as to what happened and ask why and how? God has asked us to be like children. Just because we want to know and not defy His

Word or disobey, God will add to our knowledge in the appropriate time.

> *Isaiah 14:12-15 (KJV) How art thou fallen from heaven, O Lucifer, son of the morning! How art thou cut down to the ground, which didst weaken the nations! [13] For thou hast said in thine heart, I will ascend into heaven, I will exalt my throne above the stars of God: I will sit also upon the mount of the congregation, in the sides of the north: [14] I will ascend above the heights of the clouds; I will be like the most High. [15] Yet thou shalt be brought down to hell, to the sides of the pit.*

God has given us the privilege of asking why or wondering or pondering over matters as long as we do not try to add or subtract from the Word, or, use it as stumbling blocks to others. We should also understand that answers to many of our questions would be available to us only after we depart from the world, and, even then, only in God's good time.

It is true that God has given us minds that ask why? Any one with a child knows that there is no end to the 'why's raised by the child. The parents are expected to give the right answer to help the mind of the child to grow normally. It is also very true that the parents who do not have the answers to most of the "whys" from the child get frustrated and annoyed!

In this day and age, parents are so irresponsible and unconcerned that they let their children get their questions answered at school or by some predator that gives them wrong and dangerous answers for their questions.

The present day breakdown in morality and in the families, societies, and nation are because of the parents who are too busy to mold the minds of their beloved children!

When our brains stop asking us "why?" it is an indication that our brain is dead or dying. The enquiring inquisitive mind is a basic need for a rapid learner as well as an educator. But it also can get one into trouble.

I have seen many monkeys being trapped because of their inquisitiveness. The gypsies catch their monkeys utilizing the inquisitiveness of the monkeys. I saw a documentary about a tree python climbing up a tree. All the adult monkeys ran away, but a young monkey would not heed the warning, but started to grab the python's head.

The python was not hungry, and it was only after many attempts to shake the young monkey off, that it finally obliged the monkey by catching and reluctantly swallowing it. The pathetic cries of the young monkey being squeezed to death could only evoke impotent cries from the mother monkey that had been calling the foolish offspring, playing with danger.

Knowledge is a dangerous weapon in the hands of the fools and the wicked. It can turn the head and heart of the naïve and foolish into becoming proud predators. The examples are abundant around us, among more primitive people as well as highly educated fools and fanatics.

The desire to produce more lethal weapons has eventually made wise fools look into the atom. This has led to the production of atomic and other bombs that can destroy the earth and entire mankind.

We are even now made to look into the atoms to see our potential total demise. In our lives, we will come across our children in play, barely out of their diapers, trying to stick metal pins into electrical sockets, and slightly older children try to play the game of parenting [sex].

It is the responsibility of the parent to give strict warnings to the children that such games are forbidden till the children are mature and ready, to deal with the dire consequences for satisfying their curiosity and interest without being hurt.

I tried to read up as much I could about snakes. I found that almost every country, culture, and religion around the world has had images of snakes woven into their fabric. Snakes found their place in mythology, religion, fashion, culture, trade and even diet.

There has been a global 'deification' of serpents. This follows the Biblical documentation of humanity giving in to the spiritual serpent, and the common global ancestry. Humanity has started calling good as bad, and bad as good!

In India, many worship snakes, especially the deadly cobras. They are called the "good-snake" or "Nalla Pambu". It is considered good luck and blessing if a cobra lives in the house premises!

The major gods of India are closely associated with snakes. The gods and demons were supposed to have used the serpent god Adisesha as the churning rope, while using the Himalaya Mountains as the churning spindle, with the gods on one end and the demons and giants on the other. The churning made the snake to exhale deadly venom starting to kill the demons and the gods.

One of the major gods Shiva swallowed the venom to save the other gods. His wife grabbed his throat to keep the venom from getting into Shiva's system, with the result, Shiva's face and neck turned blue.

A parallel to the Bible was presented by some scholars [Dr.Deivasigamony Ph.D.] that the present belief of people of Hindu religion is a corrupted form of Christianity, which was wide spread in India during the early centuries after Jesus.

Thomas one of the 12 disciples of Jesus and others brought Christianity. The word Shiva means love. Some of the scholars believe that the name was originally Yeshua [Jesus] who depicts the love of God. Jesus took the penalty of the sin [poison] to save those affected by sin.

The other major Hindu god is named Vishnu and is supposed to lie on the coiled body of the huge thousand-headed cobra [Adisesha] as a bed. Krishna is another major Hindu god who subdued a dangerous snake by dancing on its head and hood.

Many carvings of half human half snake are seen in many parts of India. These findings show how humanity is affiliating itself with the serpents, and adopted serpents as their deity. Five headed cobras are often seen in carvings hovering over the head to offer shade from the sun, and the five heads and the hood of the snake is to represent a gesture of benediction.

Some believe that if and when a cobra hovers over a baby with the hood spread over the baby, it will indicate that the baby will grow up to be a great leader! People have festivals every year, called the Nag Panchami when the entire town or village will catch and bring live cobras into their town, and even homes to pay them homage before returning them unharmed to the fields or forests where they caught them from.

The deification and affiliation to the serpent is seen in other countries and religions.

American Indians and the Mayans worshipped and associated fertility and rain with snakes. European psychologists associated sex, serpents, and serpigenous human sperms. This is due to their own rebellion against God and to propagate atheism and anti-God philosophies.

Ancient Egyptians worshipped cobra goddess Ejo and wore the snake emblem on the crown. Australian aborigines worshipped a rainbow snake involved in creation. Scandinavians had their share of snake worship. Greco-Roman mythology had supernatural serpents like Hydra and Medusa.

The Medical emblem called caduceus is from Roman lore, showing two twining serpents on a rod, with Mercury's wings bringing healing.

The Greek philosophy of reincarnation generated the "Ourorboros" where a serpent is seen to swallow part of its tail to project the symbol of the eternal circle or cipher. The endless circle of 'Ourorboros' was to introduce the concept of reincarnation.

The ancient Greek trade ships traded this idea to India and other countries with which it traded. All these confirm the infiltration of the satanic serpent, dominating humanity.

Chapter 7

Serpent's War on the Son

I wonder and speculate that may be Lucifer, the good-looking angel, who was heaven's music minister grew presumptuous, and started taking on himself matters not designated to him by God, and were forbidden by God.

Presumption is an arrogant uprising of 'one's -self' in rebellion. Assumption, on the other hand is often a foolish mistake. God knowing that Lucifer was still too immature to handle certain things [possibly the fruit of the tree of life] might have forbidden it. The Word [Bible] affirms that knowledge puffs one up.

1 Cor. 8:1 (KJV) Knowledge puffeth up, but charity edifieth.

Before God could give Lucifer the capacity to stomach the effects of the forbidden potent fruit, this angel might have 'bitten' the forbidden fruit from the tree of knowledge of good and evil, long before humans did. [The knowledge could have caused sinister sin mutation of his spiritual DNA and RNA, and also given Luçifer access to infect and play with the DNA and RNA of humanity to produce mutations that would bring death and separation from God. The generations of Nephelims are possible evidence to this.].

This forbidden fruit may have been a vegetable matter or a spiritual 'non-matter' that really matters [such as the **fruits** of ones labor, or of the womb, or of the spirit]. Being human and limited to the fleshly dimension, we think of fruit as high in carbohydrates, vitamins, fiber etc, which feed the flesh component of us.

Food and fruits in earth are a composite of carbohydrates, proteins, fats, minerals, and vitamins to feed the bodies of inhabitants of earth, whose bodies are out of mud, and earth. The food for the soul and the spirit are different.

The Bible addresses that the 'spirit and the soul' components consider 'fruits' as *"love, joy, peace, patience, kindness goodness, faithfulness, and self-control."* [Galatians.5:22]

> *Genesis 2:17 "but you must not eat from the tree of the knowledge of good and evil, for when you eat of it you will surely die."*

It appears as though this arrogant and presumptuous action resulted in this angel being overcome by evil to such an extent that he became Satan [the Serpent] and developed his age-old bellyaching against God. For, instead of repenting of his pride in assuming that he was equal to God, and that he also could handle good and not be affected by evil, he was completely overcome by evil. His disobedience and hurt- pride started his 'delinquent' rebellion against God Himself.

**He was once called the morning star,
but pride made him fall.**

Isaiah 14:12 "How you have fallen from heaven, O morning star, son of the dawn! You have been cast down to the earth, you who once laid low the nations!"

I continue in my mortal imagination, that Lucifer, who was the son of dawn, presumed that he was the first-born and the next in command to God Himself. He might have considered that he should be part of the Trinity of God-head, and that Jesus the God-Son should have no place in the Trinity.

Being the music minister with a large choir team, this 'rocky' music minister [who took a 'rap' in heaven,] misled a third of the angels to join him in his rebellion against their Creator. He might have thrown a challenge to God that the evil, which now controlled him, was as strong as the goodness and holiness that God represented, and was an inevitable and necessary 'balance' needed in God's creation.

He might have challenged, that God had to prove that good can prevail over evil and that 'every action needs to have an equal and opposite reaction'. He might have even made the challenge to the Son of God in particular. The Word of God says that when you treat a servant like a son, he demands to be made a son.

Proverbs 29:21 (NLT) "A servant who is pampered from childhood will later become a rebel."

Satan probably presumed that he should be treated as the first son, and that Jesus the Word of God and the Son should be considered as only the second child, and that Satan should be considered as the rightful 'heir' to God!!! Satan must have been hoping for God to die, or retire!!

We see the result of this enactment on earth through Cain the first born to humans to murder his younger brother, Abel. We experience the war of ages between the Ishmaelite (children of the elder) who want to exterminate the Israelites (children of the younger).

Later, we see the older Esau and his generation of Edomites wanted and tried to destroy Jacob and his descendants, the Israelites. We as humans are restricted by the three dimensions, [matter, space and time], and strictly confined by the 'Time' element. Except in our imagination, we are unable to travel back and forth in time. There can be no such dimensional restriction for the heavenly hosts.

Eccles. 3:15 (NLT) "Whatever exists today and whatever will exist in the future has already existed in the past. For God calls each event back in its turn."

That is why the Bible says that Jesus the Lamb of God was slain for us, even before the world and its inhabitants were created.

Chapter 8

Seduction of the Serpent

As discussed earlier, Satan wanted to be equal with God, and might have wanted to displace the Son of God from the Trinity.

The Bible says, that when the world was created, it was done jointly with the Word [the Son], though Jesus came into the world as a human many hundreds of years later than creation of Adam and Eve, and was therefore called as the Son of God and the son of mankind.

John 1:1 "In the beginning was the Word, and the Word was with God, and the Word was God. He was with God in the beginning. Through him all things were made; without him nothing was made that has been made."

God had approved of the creation and found it was good.

Gen 1:31 "God saw all that he had made, and it was very good."

This seems to have angered Satan, for he thought that when he did some thing.

['Something' which he was not supposed to do,] God would allow it to backfire [another presumption] whereas God approved the Son's work namely the creation of the earth and its inhabitants, especially the humans, and 'considered it good'.

So, he wants to discredit the Son of God by pulling down the creation on earth, to decay, and, corrupting humanity to a physical death and a permanent separation from God.

In his spirit and in his mind Satan decided to get rid of Jesus, the Son. He could not do it in the spirit realm, and planned to do it on earth, to murder Jesus the Son of God in the human form.

1] This may be the reason [probably] why the Bible calls Satan the 'murderer'.

2] For Satan's scheming plans to displace the Son of God from the Trinity and usurp the Son's heritage and obtain a placement whether in the Trinity or somewhere else, he was called the 'thief.'

3] Through his lies to discredit God, and by causing the downfall of some of the angels and all of humanity, Satan made himself into the father of 'lies.'

Chapter 9

Serpent Bites the Humans

The Word, who became the Son of God and Lord Jesus on earth, made it very clear in His teaching, that crimes such as adultery or stealing or murder, are already committed in the mind and the heart; whether or not they are followed through to a physical conclusion. For, the physical body is only a small, temporary, weak component of each complex human being.

Each one of us is made of three major parts: the body, the spirit and the soul, with input from the mind, emotion, will and conscience. Anger in the mind is murder, and it harmfully and dangerously affects the body, spirit and soul.

> *"For out of the heart come evil thoughts, murder, adultery, sexual immorality, theft, false testimony, slander."*

Mark 7:20 "He went on: 'What comes out of a man is what makes him 'unclean.' For from within, out of men's hearts, come evil thoughts, sexual immorality, theft, murder, adultery, greed, malice, deceit, lewdness, envy, slander, arrogance and folly. All these evils come from inside and make a man 'unclean.' ' "

The once morning star, wanted to seduce and corrupt the human. Satan figuratively has a three-pronged trident as his weapon. The prongs are [a] The lusts of the eyes. [b] The lusts of the flesh. [c] The pride of life.

Satan approached Eve, in the belly-slithering form, of a sinuous, sensual serpent that can enter the smallest crevice in the fence, or hedge. He tried to make God a liar, with his own twisted lies, saying:

1]   "You" meaning Eve (and Adam was indirectly included) will not die if you eat the fruit that has been forbidden. He (Satan) himself ate it and (thought that) he did not die.

Genesis 3:4 " 'You will not surely die,' the serpent said to the woman."

This was catering to the lusts of the eyes, *"and the fruit was good to look at."* What Satan still has not understood, nor wants us to know is that...

In God's sight, separation from goodness and holiness is *death*. Separation from Holiness will bring about eternal separation from the holy God.

As God is life, a life without God is death.

2]   God did not love them [Adam and Eve] like 'Himself'. So He held back from them the fruit that would make them like God.

Genesis 3:5 "For God knows that when you eat of it your eyes will be opened, and you will be like God, knowing good and evil."

This temptation is to evoke covetousness, catering to the "lusts of the flesh", wanting what some one else has, this time it is what God has.

3]   They [Eve and Adam] need not obey God if they would be equal, and they could get along without any fear of God, not feel obligated to Him, but live free from God's control!

This temptation caters to the "Pride of life"

4]   Satan has recommended that they [Adam and Eve and their progeny] should have an open mind that should question and re-evaluate matters. Just because God created humanity and told them to look after earth, and given them a free will, they need not be seeking to do God's whims and desires. Humanity should exercise their own 'Human-Rights' to stand on their own feet, and not be accountable to any body [Especially to God, otherwise, it would be no freedom!].

When children are grown up, they have to cut loose from their parents and need to live their own lives. They should consider God is only like our umbilicus. Incidentally, Adam, and Eve were created and made and not born and therefore, did not have nor needed 'the umbilicus'. Their children [of Adam and Eve] however did need them.

[Satan suggests that there is no umbilicus needed between God and humanity, only between humans and humans]. The modern philosophy is becoming, "If any thing makes you feel good, you should consider that it is good". One need not be accountable to God.

This temptation caters to the "Lusts of the flesh"

Satan probably took the first bite to encourage Eve to take the second bite from the same fruit. [Not in the Word - my personal theorizing] The following ['third'] bite was by Adam.

> Genesis 3:6 *"When the woman saw that the fruit of the tree was good for food and pleasing to the eye, and also desirable for gaining wisdom, she took some and ate it. She also gave some to her husband, who was with her, and he ate it."*

Satan focuses humanity's eyes on the transient 'erotic' In-order to cut them off from God, with things 'erratic'.

The poison of the serpent in the fruit and the ill effects of the forbidden fruit entered the bellies of human beings, and since then they also have been 'bellyaching' against God.

Since that time, mankind has had poison entering into their 'blood' [the scripture refers to blood as life], into their bodies, into their natures, into their minds, into their desires, into their spirits and, even into their souls.

Sin by separating us from the holy God, started acting like lethal mutant viruses passed from generation to generation, resulting in our moral and physical death and decay.

The mutation due to sin not only produce genetic transference of diabetes, high-blood pressure, allergies, asthma, incompetent immune system, certain cancers, mental-disorders, psychotic behaviors, afflicting our bodies, but also our emotions, behaviors and our spirits, such as anger, corruption of morals etc.

Chapter 10

Serpent's Venom Begins to Act

**Terrestrial Snakebite Affecting a Minority of Humanity
Spiritual Snakebite Affecting 100% of Humanity
in Every Generation**

It is interesting to understand the method of 'killing'. The Word says that God breathed "breath" into human nostrils to give life. When we stop breathing, we die.

The Bible says that the secret of life is in the "blood". The snake venoms, [both terrestrial and spiritual] are seen to target these two vital areas, namely: 1.The blood, and 2. The breath.

Cobras, Coral snakes, Mambas, etc are called the elapids and kill predominantly by a neuro toxin that paralyses the muscles of respiration and the higher centers that keeps us breathing whether we are awake, or asleep. The neuro toxins cause death by paralyzing our breathing muscle, and stopping our breath.

Rattlesnakes, Russell's vipers, Pit vipers etc belong to the viper group, which kills by blood poisoning- a hemo-toxin. The blood clots tend to block-off vessels supplying vital organs. The loss of the clotting ability of the blood results in oozing out of the small blood vessels in the muscles, abdominal viscous etc.

The tissues and the internal organs undergo necrosis. As the venom seeps up from the snakebite the victim experiences excruciating burning pain.

As described earlier, the poison has two major methods of killing:

1] Working like a Neuro toxin, it soon paralyzes mankind's will power as well as their sane thinking [higher-centers for breathing and heart beating]. It eventually causes 'respiratory failure' as their ability to get 'inspiration' from above [God] becomes impaired causing asphyxiation, and, the poisoned blood brings about a fatal 'heart-attack'- [death to the heart].

The nerve centers are the major areas for our cognitive [rational] thinking. The Satan's venom affects this, and people loose their value system. The educational system becomes anti-moral and anti-god. Education is transformed to perversion, and begins to pervade into all systems of communication.

2] The second method is through Hemo-toxin and necrotization. The blood going through various muscles and internal organs causes blood clotting, as well as internal bleedings and necrosis [death of] the tissue, which includes vital organs for survival.

It is Satan's poisonous purpose, to bring wickedness into all mankind, so that they show that the work [creation of earth and the human beings] of the Son of God [Word of God] was a total failure, and, that the Son is not fit to be part of God's Trinity.

The cardio-vascular system that is a sensitive indicator of our "Emotional state," begins to malfunction due to the hemo-toxins. Passions take precedence over Reason, and become perverted. Wrong Desires, Greed, Covetousness, with extreme self-centeredness, makes the hearts become erratic in rate, rhythm and function, and fails.

Instead of compassion flowing from the belly, blood oozes out of most abdominal viscous, as the normal clotting mechanism fails.

The result on humanity is a poisoned body, mind, soul, and spirit with, sickness, severe pain and death. Our only hope is through the Son, who can provide the antivenin. Just as the sun sheds light for our life application, the Son sheds His light and truth, which bring us freedom and life.

Before we had the light on the types of snake venom and the specific antitoxin, we treated people by making a criss-cross incision over the bite, squeeze out blood, or use the mouth to suck out any poison, provided there is no ulceration in the mouth, and spit it out.

Some branded the site of bite. Some put all kinds of poultice, or, broken phonographic disc. Others went to 'shamans'.

Since we are enlightened about the composition of the venom, we have started collecting the various snake venoms by manually holding the snakes and milking their venom in to a wine glass covered by thin rubber sheet.

The venom is freeze-dried. It can hold its potency for over 50 years. A tiny fraction of the venom is injected into horse, and after the horse recovers, progressively increasing doses of venom are injected into the horse, till its serum shows anti bodies against the snake venom.

Later, blood from the horse is drawn out. The serum is separated from the blood, and measured doses of the antivenin in the serum are put into vials freeze-dried and sealed. These antivenin serums will be used on humans, who have been bitten by snakes.

The Son of God is the one who created the universe, the sun and the solar system. He is also the Light that helps us to see, and learn the truth and to live.

We now have scientific proof, that when we are cut off from sunlight, the earth and its inhabitants will perish. The sun that gives light and heat is only one of God's creations. I cannot even imagine what a catastrophe it would be to be cut off from the Son of God who is the very source of our life!

Chapter 11

Antivenin Preparation against Serpent Bite

Repeating for emphasis, the [medical] snake antivenins are prepared from progressive injection of tiny amounts of a variety of snake venom into a horse and getting the horse serum antivenin.

My brother Samuel Johnson was in King Institute, Chennai [Madras] in charge of supervising venom extraction from snakes and other venomous creatures, and preparing antivenin by injecting tiny doses into horses. This is a dangerous work, and the team is aware that their efforts are worth the risk because of the vast number of people whose lives may be saved by the anti-venom. I had the opportunity of studying this aspect too.

The first step is to catch the different types of cobras, vipers and kraits, alive and milk their venom into a glass or plastic container

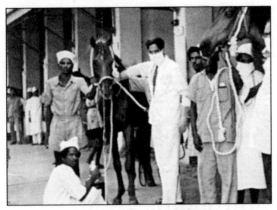

Dr. Samuel Johnson of the team
in the King Institute, Guindy.

with a wide mouth, covered up by a membrane or rubber sheet. The snakes are returned to their natural habitat, or kept in a special cage or an enclosure well protected, from where they can be caught again and again for milking more venom.

A tribal group called 'Irrullas' in South India seems to handle snakes unusually well and don't die like others by snakebites.

They are a great help to the larger institutes and individual trying to catch snakes. The milked venom is quick frozen and preserved. Tiny amounts of the venom are injected into healthy horses. Over a period, the horses develop anti bodies to the venom. The horse's blood is drawn, the antibodies in the serum is separated and sterilized, 'quantitated', put into vials to be injected into victims of snakebite. Specific snake venoms produce specific antibodies.

Some centers try to get a mixed antivenin to treat people who do not know what type of snake bit them. In general, the cobra venom is predominantly neuro-toxic and viper venom hemo-toxic, but many of them have mixed venom.

India gets its supply of antivenin from Haffkine Institute Bombay. Each country depends on their national antivenin institutes. Some of the victim may die from allergic-anaphylactic reaction to the antivenin to horse/animal allergy. Some die due to inadequate dose of antivenin, and others as the venom was of a different type, or due to delay in administration.

The omniscient, omnipresent and omnipotent Triune God was aware of the problem of Satan's sabotage coming up, even during the time of creation, and the Son was prepared. We the humans are limited by 'time' and have three segments of time as 'past, present and future'. But God is not limited to or by our 'time'. As mentioned earlier, that is why the Lamb of God was slain as a sacrifice on our behalf, before we were even created.

The antivenin prepared and offered by God had no anaphylactic dangers and is effective against every kind of venom of the spiritual serpents.

All that is required is to seek the antivenin in time. As God Himself offers it, during our lifetime, there is no transport delay or insufficient supply of the antivenin.

It has been prepared from an eternal Lamb. It is interesting to learn that on terra, [on earth] there are efforts to use sheep instead of horse for preparing antivenin.

*Revelation 13:8 "All inhabitants of the earth will worship the beast—all whose names have not been written in the book of life belonging to **the Lamb that was slain from the creation of the world**."*

Jesus offered to become a human person, vulnerable to all the weaknesses of human being. He was willing to be bitten by this venomous serpent Satan with the most deadly venom called as sin, carrying with it the final sting called as death and decay.

Yes there was a catch. If Jesus gave into sin in any way, He would not have been able to produce antibodies in His Blood against sin, death and Satan in-order to save us human beings. That was the reason Satan tried to kill Jesus when He was a child through King Herod. Later, Satan tempted Jesus in every way possible; starting from the time Jesus started His ministry with a forty-day fasting.

Many of the disciples succumbed to Satan and were used to get Jesus to fault or falter. Finally Satan worked on "Religion" and religious leaders to kill Jesus within three years of starting of His ministry, hoping to nip it in the 'bud'. But it was the serpent at the root of this action. Thus Jesus was able to die as the sinner's substitute, and offer His sinless sacred Blood as 'antivenin'.

God was aware of Satan's fall. Because of His great love that has no boundaries, God wants to make a way to overcome the evil let loose by Satan and his minions. Yet, God is holy and just. He cannot overlook evil and sin, which have nature's 'built-in penalties'. These

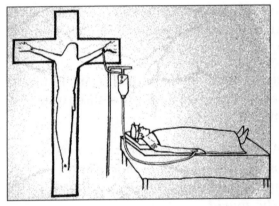

penalties separate our spirits from God's Holy Spirit: our bodies become corrupt, decayed, and diseased, to decease [die] and even our souls that sin, die.

The Son of God volunteered to pay for the penalty of the fallen and corrupt humanity, making a way for humanity to be restored to a sinless eternity with God, if during our life we repent, seek God's forgiveness, forsake our wicked ways and receive the gift of new life offered through His self sacrifice. This fact as a prophecy was openly declared in Isaiah, Chapter 53, written almost seven hundred years before Jesus was born.

Isaiah 53:3-11 "He was despised and rejected by men; a man of sorrows, and familiar with suffering. Like one from whom men hide their faces he was despised, and we esteemed him not.

*Surely he took up our infirmities and carried our sorrows;
yet we considered him stricken by God, smitten by him, and
afflicted.*

*But he was pierced for our transgressions, he was crushed
for our iniquities; the punishment that brought us peace
was upon him, and by his wounds we are healed.*

*We all, like sheep, have gone astray, each of us has turned
to his own way; and the LORD has laid on him the iniquity
of us all.*

*He was oppressed and afflicted, yet he did not open his
mouth; he was led like a lamb to the slaughter and as a
sheep before her Shearer's is silent, so he did not open his
mouth.*

*By oppression and judgment he was taken away. And who
can speak of his descendants? For he was cut off from the
land of the living; for the transgression of my people he
was stricken.*

*He was assigned a grave with the wicked and with the rich
in his death, though he had done no violence, nor was any
deceit in his mouth.*

*Yet it was the Lord's will to crush him and cause him to
suffer, and though the LORD makes his life a guilt offering,
he will see his offspring and prolong his days, and the will
of the LORD will prosper in his hand.*

*After the suffering of his soul, he will see the light of life and
be satisfied; by his knowledge my righteous servant will
justify many, and he will bear their iniquities.*

Satan, can read and quote the Scriptures, but cannot understand
the 'Word' the embodiment of the Scriptures. So Satan interprets the
mercy of God as a weakness in the Trinity, which he should be able to
exploit.

John 3:16, "For God so loved the world that he gave his only Son, so that everyone who believes in him will not perish but have eternal life."

Satan thought that he could eliminate the Son of God in His "human form" and get into the position of authority held by the Son in the Trinity. Jesus even told this as a parable, not only to the Pharisees, but also to us.

Matthew 21:38-39 "But when the tenants saw the son, they said to each other, 'This is the heir. Come, let's kill him and take his inheritance.' So they took him and threw him out of the vineyard and killed him."

Luke 20:13-15 "Then the owner of the vineyard said, 'What shall I do? I will send my son, whom I love; perhaps they will respect him.'

But when the tenants saw him, they talked the matter over. 'This is the heir,' they said. 'Let's kill him, and the inheritance will be ours.' So they threw him out of the vineyard and killed him. What then will the owner of the vineyard do to them?"

Could this be a remote explanation for God's elect?

God had forbidden physical relation between the flesh [humans] and the spirit world. Necromancy, divination and spirit-medium contacts are forbidden in the Bible.

Jesus told us this important principle when questioned by the scribes, "that there is no sex in heaven, or marriages."

Matt. 22:30 (KJV) "For in the resurrection they neither marry, nor are given in marriage, but are as the angels of God in heaven."

Satan tries to defy God in every way possible. Therefore, there are recorded cases of "demon possession of humans" and, "demonic intercourse's with humans". Some authors have recorded sexual orgies not only between humans because of our own wickedness, but also between evil spirits and humans, to produce polluted, mutated offspring.

I do not know for certain about the validity of this, but it makes me wonder if there is a possibility [Reader, be aware that the Word of God does not mention it, and it is only my speculation] that Satan not only entered the mind of Eve to seduce her, but could he have seduced her body also?

And could such be the reason for the very first born on earth to have become a murderer of his younger brother for a relatively trivial cause, and that too, due to anger that was directed against God [as his personal offering was turned down in favor of the one from his brother].

1 John 3:12 refers to Cain saying, "...who was of that wicked one." Not as Cain, who was of that wicked one, and slew his brother. And wherefore slew he him? Because his own works were evil, and his brother's righteous.

This idea that Satan could have seduced Eve's body may be revolting to many (even to me). But every one would agree that when our mind and spirit are seduced, the result was, and still is the same, as having been done in our body, as the body is only an extension of our psyche the mind to influence our souls.

Matthew 5:28 "But I say unto you, that whosoever looketh on a woman to lust after her hath committed adultery with her already in his heart."

Chapter 12

Snake
Venom
Wipes
Out
Many
People

Angels though they are spirits, have been documented in the scripture to materialize and bear offspring with humans. This physical cohabitation of the spirits and human resulted in wicked, violent people and was one of the causes of the great global flood of Noah's time.

I do not believe that every bad person has been spawned of the demons physically, and that they are the 'non-elect' mentioned in the Word. But I believe that even though we were made in the image of the Holy God, Satan, as well as our own sin, has destroyed all our human spirits, and that **it does not make any great difference**

whether the [soma] bodies of women have been assaulted
and raped by the evil spirits while their minds have already
been. The result is the same, namely, separation from the
Holy God.

> 1 John 3:12 **"Do not be like Cain, who belonged to
> the evil one** and murdered his brother. And why did he
> murder him? Because his own actions were evil and his
> brother's were righteous."

> Genesis 6:4 "The Nephilim were on the earth in those days—
> and also afterward—when the sons of God went to the
> daughters of men and had children by them." [Forbidden
> Act]

> Matthew 13:24-30 "Jesus told them another parable: "The
> kingdom of heaven is like a man who sowed good seed in
> his field. But while everyone was sleeping, his enemy came
> and sowed weeds among the wheat, and went away. When
> the wheat sprouted and formed heads, then the weeds also
> appeared. The owner's servants came to him and said, **'Sir,
> didn't you sow good seed in your field? Where
> then did the weeds come from?'**

> **'An enemy did this,' he replied.** The servants asked
> him, 'Do you want us to go and pull them up?' 'No,' he
> answered, 'because while you are pulling the weeds, you
> may root up the wheat with them. **Let both grow
> together until the harvest. At that time I will tell
> the harvesters: First collect the weeds and tie them
> in bundles to be burned; then gather the wheat
> and bring it into my barn.' " "**

> Matthew 13:37 "He answered, 'The one who sowed the
> good seed is the Son of Man.' "

Matthew 13:38-40 "The field is the world, and the good seed stands for the sons of the kingdom. The weeds are the sons of the evil one, and the enemy who sows them is the devil. The harvest is the end of the age, and the harvesters are angels. As the weeds are pulled up and burned in the fire, so it will be at the end of the age."

Chapter 13

Self-Destructive Serpent and His Slaves

These above passages may explain **why though we all are called, only a few are chosen.**

The venom of the serpent will kill unless the antivenin is administered in time. Is it not an unexplainable stupidity that causes humans, bitten by the serpent to reject and refuse the freely offered treatment?

Though Satan could read the scriptures, because he himself is a liar and evil, he could not believe that God would be so open and naively honest. He also trusts that if he, a powerful spirit, can reject the love of God; he could control a good number of the weak humans also to reject help from God [The Bible says, that unless God opens the 'willing' heart, the eyes may see and the ears may hear, but the mind would not understand the truth].

Isaiah 44:18 "Such stupidity and ignorance! Their eyes are closed, and they cannot see. Their minds are shut, and they cannot think."

Luke 18:34 [even] "The disciples did not understand any of this. Its meaning was hidden from them, and they did not know what he was talking about."

Chapter 14

The
Fool
is
Taken
in his
own Snare

Satan really played into God's plan of salvation for mankind by pushing Jesus to His death on the cross, within three years of His ministry, and when he was barely 33 years old. He thought foolishly and arrogantly, that by getting the Lord Jesus crucified by the humanity He came to save, would somehow alienate God and humanity forever. But he could not understand the real Love of God, having severed himself from God voluntarily.

Satan perceived the love of God to be God's weakness. For, when Satan and a group of his team rebelled against God, (who was the all powerful creator of himself and the other rebelling angels,) God did not destroy them at once. And though Isaiah prophesied that he would be thrown down into perdition, God had not still banished Satan from the heaven, the kingdom of God. For, Satan with his team went to challenge God about Job, the faithful human servant of God.

> *Job 1:6-12 (NLT) One day the angels came to present themselves before the Lord, and Satan the Accuser came with them. [7] "Where have you come from?" the Lord asked Satan. And Satan answered the Lord, "I have been going back and forth across the earth, watching everything that's going on."*
>
> *[8] Then the Lord asked Satan, "Have you noticed my servant Job? He is the finest man in all the earth—a man of complete integrity. He fears God and will have nothing to do with evil."*
>
> *[9] Satan replied to the Lord, "Yes, Job fears God, but not without good reason! [10] You have always protected him and his home and his property from harm. You have made him prosperous in everything he does. Look how rich he is! [11] But take away everything he has, and he will surely curse you to your face!"*
>
> *[12] "All right, you may test him," the Lord said to Satan. "Do whatever you want with everything he possesses, but don't harm him physically." So Satan left the Lord's presence.*

Later, he petitioned to 'sift' Simon Peter the impulsive disciple of Jesus, just before Jesus was ready to take upon Him the sin of humanity and die on the Cross for humanity. Lord Jesus offered to become the advocate (defense counsel) for Peter, and later, for all of us.

> *Luke 22:31-32 (NLT) "Simon, Simon, Satan has asked to have all of you, to sift you like wheat. [32] But I have pleaded in prayer for you, Simon that your faith should not fail. So when you have repented and turned to me again, strengthen and build up your brothers."*

Chapter 15

The Serpent Bites The Savior

Satan thought that though Jesus was the Word of God, in the flesh, while carrying humanity's sin as a human, He could be got rid of. Being the almighty God, who created the human race, Jesus was able to be born as a human without the requirement of sex, for Satan had corrupted all flesh.

[Satan remembered that he could really control the Nephilim to aggravate humanity to gross rebellion, sin and violence, and though Jesus was born through the Holy Spirit of God, Jesus had to be a human through a woman to be acceptable to the humans. Satan felt that he could manipulate humanity as he pleased and that he could take-on JESUS IN A HUMAN FORM, HUMAN SETTING WITH THE HUMAN LIMITATIONS.]

Jesus COMPLETED God's will and Purpose, breaking humanity free from their voluntary slavery to Satan. What more, He promised to send to us the Holy Spirit in His place, not only as a comforter, but **also to empower us to receive a new birth in the spirit**. The Holy Spirit, when we are willing and cooperative will mould us and present us faultless before the presence of the glory of God.

Jesus did not break God's own rules, and sex did not play any roll in the birth of Jesus. Nor does sex play any part, in the 'rebirth' offered to us to obtain a restored eternal life with God.

On earth we see three major groups of humanity. One group hates God and any thing and any one standing for morality or holiness. They are self-pleasers, and Satan pleasers.

The second group seeks God, and wants to please God.

The third larger group just gropes around double minded in all things, including finding out where they are headed for an eternal future.

Jesus said that God plants good seeds in the soil. But Satan comes in the night to plant weeds, either poisonous or parasitical to suck out the nourishment from the soil, to keep it from the plants growing from the good seeds.

The weeds may represent the 'Non-elect' who take after their father the devil. But, God's love is so great, that He offers His salvation to them also. He offers to graft even the wild wines to Himself so that they may yield good fruits.

Romans 11:23-24 (KJV) "And they also, if they abide not still in unbelief, shall be graffed in: for God is able to graff them in again.

[24] For if thou wert cut out of the olive tree which is wild by nature, and wert graffed contrary to nature into a good olive tree: how much more shall these, which be the natural branches, be graffed into their own olive tree?"

Satan the serpent repeatedly tried to bite Jesus – i.e. at the beginning of His ministry, after His fasting prayer, with three cunning temptations, using the scriptures. Later Satan made His disciples deny, and even betray Him.

When God's time was ripe, in the Garden of Gethsemane, Jesus offered to be bitten by all the spiritual serpents' venom in order to give His blood for humanity for preparation as the one and only antivenin. It was done with great agony as it put the entire sin of humanity on Him.

Though He committed no sin, He was made into sin and had to die to pay the penalty of sin. From then, and His death within a few hours and three days, He was cut off from His communion and connection with God the Father who had to stay Holy and just.

Satan was ecstatic. He had Jesus falsely tried [? six times], had Him whipped and tortured almost to death, hoping to evoke anger or any form of retaliation, which Satan thought would put Jesus in his power and annul His effort to salvage the human race.

But the Lord Jesus went through His ordeal patiently, and with no diminution of His love for us sinners.

For, even as He was upon the cross, He cried: "Father, forgive them, for they know not what they do". Thus He crowned His work of bringing hope for us, the humans lost in the poisonous toxic effects of sin.

Chapter 16

The
Son
Survives
and
Revives
Victims

Though Jesus willingly offered to pay the penalty for all sinners, he did agonize because, of the enormous ugliness of sin. That which He took upon Himself was totally alien to His nature.

We see only a glimpse of this agony in His prayer at the garden of Gethsemane, where despite the cool of the hour, His sweat drops fell as great drops of blood.

He could have cancelled His offer to go to the cross even at this point, but His commitment was total and sincere. He agonized again when He was upon the cross as our sin separated Him briefly from the

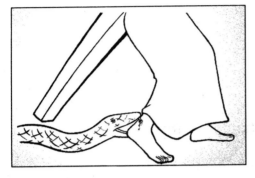

Holy Father God from whom he had been never separated, even from before creation, evoking the cry 'Father, why have you forsaken me'.

This was, I believe, is the moment when the Father had to let go the Son's hand to allow the Son to gather the sinner's hands to put them into God's holy hands, restoring the relationship between God and us.

Jesus allowed Himself to be bitten in the heel by the serpent to produce 'anti-sin-venom' and died a human death, for, <u>death is the built-in penalty of sin.</u>

Genesis 3:15 "And I will put enmity between you and the woman, and between your offspring and hers; he will crush your head, and you will strike his heel."

Chapter 17

Your Choice - The Savior or the Serpent

Jesus could have crushed the serpent's head before the serpent could bite His heel. He did not do so for two reasons. One was to give even to the serpent an opportunity to have a self-confrontation and change.

The main reason was He knew that the serpent will not repent, but will bite Him to kill Him. The purpose for which Jesus came down from heaven was to develop antivenin from His own sinless blood for the sinners in the world dying because of snake poison in their body.

Though Jesus died for sinners, His pure, uncorrupted blood could not be poisoned by sin of self or Satan. He produced heavenly antibodies in His blood against the most venomous snake poison namely, sin.

So He offered His blood to bring life and recovery to those who have been bitten by the snake and had sin poisoning their blood. **This blood with antivenin shed for all humanity is now available to you and me.**

2 Corinthians 5:21 "God made him who had no sin to be sin for us, so that in him we might become the righteousness of God."

The physical death of Jesus was offered to ensure us that our physical death brought about by the corruption in and around us need not be the end of us.

Jesus rose up from death and ascended up to heaven, assuring us that He will also take our spirits and souls to be with Him into eternity.

When Adam and Eve were created, they were given the opportunity to live forever. God warned them about the fruit of knowledge of handling good and evil, for the 'evil' would overcome them, and kill them.

God wanted mankind to be pure and innocent, but not ignorant. Mankind rebelled, and broke the only restraint God had placed on them. They broke their faith with God and in listening to Satan, considered and treated the holy God as a liar and a cheat!

Serpent's Sneak Strikes during Death Throes

Many stinging insects, even after they are dead, can harm a person as their sting and poison get embedded into the victim. A spitting cobra, even after its neck is broken, can spit venom into any one approaching it, blinding them or even killing them. The decapitated head of a snake may still bite!

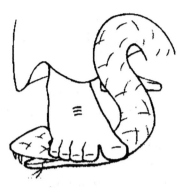

Remember Satan is not only called the murderer, he is also the father of lies. He not only spawned human murder, but later, when he found that Jesus offered the way of life into eternity for humans, he spawned another big lie called the 'evolution' of humanity. Like the venom-spitting cobra, he is spitting this lie into the eyes of some so-called educationists and stupid, lying, pseudo-scientist, who, out of curiosity, got too close to the serpent, or tried to handle it. Many of them have been blinded, but still want to be our teachers and leaders! **How ironic for the blind to insist on leading the blind!**

The purpose: The serpent wants to discredit 'creation' in the eyes of created humanity so that they would refuse to repent, and continue to blaspheme God the Creator, and lose their second opportunity of receiving salvation and eternal life through the Son of God.

Romans 6:23 *"For the wages of sin is death, but the gift of God is eternal life in Christ Jesus our Lord."*

Satan knows that humans bicker over, filter out, expose and punish small lies, but are eager to swallow big lies 'hook, line and sinker'. He knows that any gullible human believing in evolution as a fact, would consider God's Creation a myth.

This would give them the excuse that there is no God, and that they could reject the Word of God as a lie. If humans believed that they evolved from filthy primordial ooze, to cells, insects, worms etc to becoming warlords and technological wizards and demigods, then they would consider sin as only a relative term, and goodness and morality would be trashed as out-fashioned foolishness.

For evolution means only the strongest are meant to survive and the rest are to be 'food' for the survivors!

The act of various forms of physical, emotional, relational, moral aggression, violence and or even cannibalism would not be considered barbaric but quite fitting.

I wonder if any of the evolutionist ever considered that most of the protein food consumed the world over consists of the evolutionist's uncles, aunts, and grand-uncles, conveniently called beef, pork, chicken, fish, if his or her mental-midget theory were to be true!

It boggles the mind of any honest thinker how the serpent-venom could still continue to be devil and be fog us humans so easily into such absurdities and self-destructive ways!

In this presentation, we have looked at the serpent, not just as the created reptilian snakes, but as the anti- God demonic being, and the role of the evils of sin, which acts like the most toxic venom of the most venomous serpent.

Satan can be blamed only for part of the wickedness and the rest is due to the 'self' and the deep selfishness in us. Moses the precursor of Jesus was asked by God to lift-up brazen serpents for the Israelites in the desert to see and recognize, what was really killing them.

First, the serpent-bitten people had to identify the cause of their affliction. They had to become aware and acknowledge truthfully which species of serpent or serpents bit them [what specific sin]. This applies to us even to this day.

The right type of antivenin has to be administered. Every sin such as murder, adultery, stealing, lying, murmuring, ingratitude, backbiting are but a few examples of serpent bites. When the victim does not hide or cover up or give excuses, God can treat the victim.

We also need to avoid playing with the venomous serpent- sin after being treated [restored and saved]. For the serpent can bite you again.

It is necessary to admit each bite of sin, confess each sin, repent, be willing to be healed, make restitution in the manner God requires of you, and be willing to be kept from further sinning. God will take care of the rest of your recovery and protect you.

Section V

Chapter 18

The Choice of Security or Cemetery is Yours

There are numerous cures offered for poisonous snakebites around the world.

But unless the right antivenin is given in time, death will over take the victim.

You can deny saying that there are no spiritual venomous snakes on earth.

75

You may be an ardent defender of the ECCO system and protect venomous vermin from the victimized humans at all costs

Keeping mongoose and ridding the home and garden from rats may keep some snakes off, though it does not apply to all the snakes on earth.

You may have developed a fatal fascination for venomous spiritual serpents.

You may be having a death wish upon yourself.

You can choose death for this and the future life.

Or

You may choose to call on God to give you the one and only antivenin and live forever.

To put it irreverently, take the Jesus Juice, the Elixir of Eternal life right now for cure and prophylaxis against serpent bites.

There is nothing except the Cross of Jesus to keep spiritual serpent away from biting us a second time.

Jesus has brought glory to God who declared that evil can be over-come only by good. He also made it possible for the mercy, justice, pity, and love of God, for the undeserving to become 'applicable' into an acceptable form called GRACE.

May it please God that all of us, will repent and ask for, and receive, His gift of new life here on earth now, and then into eternity.

Chapter 19

The
Cross

The Crossing of the Two Crosses in the Scripture:
The Old Testament and the New Testament

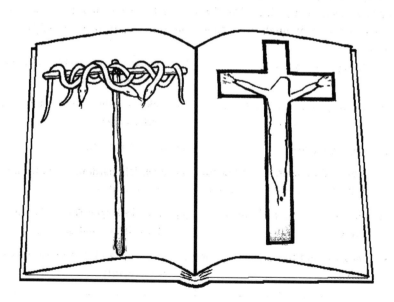

Old Testament	New Testament
Moses lifted up this brass serpent [symbol of sin and Satan] so that God's people will know what had bitten them and causing them to die – sin. Snake the symbol of sex. Snake the symbol of sensuousness. Snake the symbol of forked tongue that carries and picks up smells and stories. Snake whose mouth carries venom and death. Snake that keeps changing its skin. Snake that won't move on a straight path. Old Testament lifts up the reason [sin] which CAUSES our death and damnation so that we can	God allowed Jews and Romans to lift up Jesus. Jesus who brought God's love. Jesus who brought God's mercy. Jesus who bought pardon for each one of us. Jesus who offered Himself as sacrifice. Jesus who brought salvation and eternal life. Jesus who gave up all He could. Jesus who brought peace and joy in His mouth and life. New-Testament lifts up the Crucified Lord Jesus Christ, who is our CURE for not only sin, and death; but also the provider of our Eternal life
1] Recognize sin.	1] Recognize sin (yours) that put Jesus on the cross.
2] Acknowledge sin (confess).	2] Acknowledge your part and confess them.
3] Repent for Sin.	3] Repent for sin.
4] Seek healing from sin and death from the true expert physician.	4] Seek His pardon. Seek healing and salvation.
5] Those who did so, looked up lived.	5] If you look up at Him and believe; you will live and be saved.
6] Look up and live ±40 years on earth.	6] Look up and live victoriously for eternity.

Prayer

Holy and almighty God, I find myself sin-sick in every part of my being. I have been bitten by many sins. I identify each, ––– for none of them are hidden from your sight. I confess each, ––––one by one, ––– and repent deeply, –––––––for these sins caused the Lord Jesus to be crucified in my place. I give no excuse for any of my sins. I realize I deserve death and hell, but I pray for your mercy and undeserved grace. Wash me, cleanse, forgive, heal and save me. Give me a new life to live for You. Help me to make whatever restitution You want me to, and make me a witness to Your love, obey and glorify Your holy name.

Savior, Save Me from the Serpent and Myself.

Let my life be lived in absolute humility, in gratitude to You. Give me Your love to love other people who, like me, have been bitten by sin, and share Your love with them. Help me to hate sin that grieves You, and enable me to serve and please You, all through my life. Again I pray 'Protect me from my 'self' and from Satan'.

I humbly ask this in the name of the Lord Jesus, who gave His life for me. Amen.

Chapter $\boxed{20}$

My Personal story of deliverance from multiple, lethal snake bites

This is my story, and, this is my song,
Now I am sorry, for I had been wrong.

The Story of a deserting soldier's failure, And, yet, that of his self-sacrificing Savior.

I had been an academic 'Radiologist' most of my adult life, interested mainly in learning and confining myself to my medical specialty - 'my calling' as I called it.

I was born to Christian parents in India, who were dedicated Christians. Christians comprise less than 3% of Christians in India. I was baptized, confirmed and was professing Christianity as my religion.

At the age of sixteen, when I was a college student, I came to the understanding that my physical-birth into a Christian family did not automatically make me into a Christian!

It was a shock to come to the knowledge that to be called a Christian; every person had to come to the Cross and get to know Jesus as his or her personal Savior and to become a disciple under the personal supervision of Jesus!

Christianity is not a religion one can belong to, but is a personal relationship with the Lord Jesus.

I realized that people of every religion in the world should know that it was only the Lord Jesus who came to save sinners, and, personally paid for each sinner who comes to Him for forgiveness.

It was Jesus who shed His own blood, as He gave up His mortal life as a sin penalty in our place. He will break the power of death over the souls who seek Him. For, He rose up from death, to offer to those forgiven, an eternal life with Him. But my head knowledge of this did not make me, or any one else, a Christian.

Christianity is purely a personal relationship with Jesus and a 'follow-ship' of Jesus.

When I realized that Christ loved me so much that He suffered and died for me, I understood and was convicted that I was a miserable sinner. Then I repented and confessed my sins; making whatever restitution God put on my heart to do. Though it meant humbling my self to go and ask my enemies to forgive me, accept my guilt to authorities and others, returning stolen property, and risking punishment, these actions gave me freedom.

However, it was not any of my actions, but it was completely through His infinite mercy and grace, that I was received by the Lord Jesus, and was **born-again, born for the second time, this time,** in my spirit.

As a voluntary follower of Jesus, I was enlisted in God's army. I was proud and happy to belong to such an elite company. Incidentally, there are no civilians on earth. There are two armies at war. One is God's; under the leadership of Jesus, and the enemy army is Satan's, who is aptly named as the eternal lethal 'Serpent'.

ENLISTED IN THE ARMY

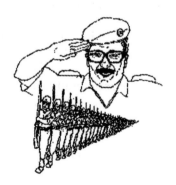

Metaphorically, and for all practical purposes, there are no civilians on the earth. There are two armies constantly at war, globally on earth, at the present 'time-span'. The army of God stands for good, but the army of the 'serpent- devil' for evil.

If we do not make a voluntary choice to seek admission in to God's army, we will automatically be dragged and forcibly enlisted into the Serpent's army. This unavoidable situation [to stay neutral] makes us all into soldiers. Therefore, to which side, we belong, is what really matters.

Armies have three components: the air force, the Navy and the ground force. The training and duties assigned to each varies. Though the functions may vary, have apparently different and diverse apparels, are still cohesive, and have an overall single purpose under God's will and authority.

Every enlisting soldier is expected to relinquish his or her personal decisions and actions, and be willing to obey orders unquestioningly, even to the extent of marching, or sailing, or of flying into a war that may maim, or kill him or her.

It is true that God offers eternal life with Him for His soldiers of His army, similar to retirement and pension benefits. But He does not offer provisions for any of the soldiers to take up matters into their own hands, nor that is the war going to be an easy one.

Jesus the Son of God had to face torture and death, and we need to be the followers of our leader Jesus.

Every person and procedure in an army should be regimented, supervised, and controlled by the will and order of God, transmitted through proper channels.

Having been born in a Christian family with my great-great grand father blessed to be a Christian convert, an evangelist and a pioneer Tamil-Christian poet, [Vedanayagam Sastriar], I presumed that I was pedigree stuff!

But, God used many others who I thought were less capable, more often and more effectively. I was annoyed and started to sulk.

The fact was that I was not willing to undergo the total submission; discipline and training the others had placed themselves in, did not register with me.

My resentful attitude and jealousy soon led me to rebellion. My resistance to discipline, lack of humility, and disobedience in the army environment actually amounts to indiscipline, open to court-martial.

I thought I already had enough stuff in me to make me a leader, not just a follower! I would say to myself that 'It is better to be the **head of a live donkey** than to be the tail of a dead tiger'. This pride probably was the start of the Serpent's rebellion, and he was casting the same net over me.

In an army, or church, or a team, one person's rebellion and foolishness can adversely or seriously endanger others. No individual can become a one-man army [as deceptively depicted by Hollywood], but, one individual can betray or weaken an entire army.

**Don't let your personal gain
Be made on another's pain**

In an army this selfish rebellious attitude causes degradation of cohesive teamwork! My pride made me loose sight of the truth, that, to be a Christian, one has **to follow Christ and not lead!**

I did not want to accept that my captain **Jesus had a servant's heart, and that was to be my discipline and training.**

But, my 'head' had become '*mulish*' by my own choice, followed by the rest of me. I would like to expose some of the seductive traps the Serpent set for me to hypnotize and get me into its sinister coils. This information may help others to avoid these landmines planted by the enemy.

There are seven stage enemy deployment maneuvers to seduce and sabotage and isolate the soldiers of God's army. These factors are applicable in our daily living, and I found this out rather late in my life. Pre warned should help you to be forearmed.

I would like to expose some of the enemy strategies, which he used effectively on me.

Deception:

One is made to feel that he/she is highly capable and should have been given more importance or, rank, rather than mere low level, mundane work. This idea seldom fails to tickle the individual's vanity!

Dilution:

Now, other worldly ambitions and pride start entering one, creating a breach in the defense within the individual. Gradual dilutions of the moral principles occur due to a process of osmosis as worldly things start to percolate inward.

Diffusion:

Good and Godly principles insidiously diffuse out, and percolate-out through the porous defense [holes in the armor].

Desiccation: [loss of moisture]

As good principles ooze out, one is left with no discipline, no obedience, loss of love for God, for fellow soldiers, and others; the army is trying to save from the Serpent. What is left of the rebel now is 'sucked out' to leave an inspissated [thick, gummy] 'self desiccated in despair.'

For, along with the loss of moisture of the love of God, also goes-out faith and hope in God.

Desperation:

When hope is lost, the situations now turn hopeless. Like a drowning person, one gropes at anything that may 'lift-one-up'. Drugs, alcohol, nicotine, sex, fame, name, violence, murder and suicide are sought, but bring no peace.

Disillusion and Desolation:

Like King Solomon did, one realizes whatever ambitions or achievements one accomplished or fulfilled, they are worthless compared to what one lost.

One realizes that one who leaves the **'Substance'** to chase the **'shadows'** find only disillusion driving one into deep Depression. Whatever one grabs to get a 'lift' or 'hype', drags one further down into guilt, shame and utter 'Destitution'. Success turns sour and insipid.

Destruction:

There may be a late realization of total loss with resultant Dissipation and Destruction of one's given lifetime. The natural principal of retribution of life lived, takes its toll on the health of the body, mind and emotions. Any one trying to jump off a high-rise building without assistance will pay with the principle of gravitation factor. One's despairs drives in psychotic transformations and destruction of one's soul and the Spirit.

These steps are the normal sequence, for every one who belongs to or captured by Serpent's army. I am sharing this, information with other soldiers in God's army so that the enemy need not take them in.

If what I have I don't share,
It is because I don't care

I will illustrate seven deadly 'D's as they happened to us in different variations, in different shapes and sizes, so watch out and keep your eyes on the Leader.

Attention trap, Scowl at Sin.

A frequently used technique by Satan to trap God's soldiers is to put on different kinds of **'Road-side' free sin-shows** as the army of God marches on. Any soldier who does not look forward but turns his eyes to see the sideshow will become the enemy's target.

Satan has a sequence of acts to hook the soldier. He **first gets the soldier's attention, even,** by making him angry and **'scowl' at** the sin show. He makes the soldier feel that he himself is above the disgusting theme, and the sideshow.

From reading the earlier portions of this book, you will recognize that I get attracted to roadside free shows. It was the earthly serpents, which caught my **Attention.**

The serpent tries all methods to get our attention. That is the start.

When I came to USA to live, I saw the tremendous technology advancement. In India, I had a SLR camera and a 16mm movie camera, as I was interested in audio-visual teaching tools. The T.V. shows in color were fascinating. Samantha the cute white witch with her bumbling husband in the show 'Bewitched' caught my attention, as did many others. Then came the show "I Love Genie," where the sexy genie goes in and out of a jar with her master who is also her boyfriend and a soldier.

During this time America was a materialistic nation, which did not believe in spirits or witches, and it was a spoof. They were on the surface light innocent comedies for laughs.

Seduction by Sin [the Serpent]

If the soldier-is 'turned-off' by the sin of the act, he will desist watching the filthy side sin show and march-on, following his Lord, to engage in battle against the source of the enemy's force.

Every soldier of God is expected to love the victims [sinners] of the enemy and tolerate and care for them.

But every soldier has to fight against the wicked principles [sin] of the enemy, and not be tolerant to sin, however mild or funny it may seem.

If any soldier does not understand this basic principle, he is fighting not for the triumph of a good and a Godly cause, but for his own ulterior motive, which is bound to be disastrous.

My gradual progression was to watch 'Newly married' marriage breaking T.V. shows and games offering rewards for the participants and laughter for the audience. The questions were to make the mates tell what the other half will do. This usually ended up with the fight between the 'newly-weds'.

It is true that God wants us to have
compassion upon sinners,
But to each, He has to give a commission
to become winners.

But, if the soldier gets angry with the people 'acting-out' a show, or, starts to 'watch' the show, he [the soldier] will become compromised. Anger is Satan's [The spiritual serpent's] remote tool, and he will use it to bring hatred or pride into the soldier. He would have already infiltrated [breached] the soldier's emotions by getting the soldier's attention to the serpent's sensational stimuli.

He will trick the soldier [you and I] into stepping off the marching column of the army to express [your and my] an objection. To do that the soldier has to believe that he has become an objective observer.

This strikes a parallel chord with my going after Balu the snake 'swallower', to study the way he was able to do what he did. I was content that this time, I was only applying my own scientific observation. I was not going after an open sin.

The soldier may see a man easing himself on the roadside, or people quarrelling on the curb. The soldier is not supposed to step off from his march to settle the problem on the roadside. The soldier's duty and objective is to stay with the army, and work as one unit, unless commissioned by the Leader, who, then will provide adequate back up.

If the soldier does step off, he has no concept, or is in contempt of being the 'defender of his country'. His action will result in choosing to end up as a street brawler, or a sanitary roadside janitor. To be a street patroller or street sweeper is not bad by itself, but it is not what the soldier of the Royal service of God is called to be doing. The army is meant for a more pressing duty.

Soldiers, who look ahead while marching,
have a destination;
Those who look around at sideshows
suffer bad fascination.

Self-decisions are Sin commission, Not for Soldiers.

If any soldier, due any reason including curiosity or good intentions [to put a stop to an unequal quarrel or to help] steps out of the ranks even **briefly, without the permission of the Leader** will find out soon what it all about. He is already entrapped. Instead of being part of the victorious army of God, he will be headed towards becoming a street brawler or a janitor on the sidewalk, with no end in sight, except that he will become a prisoner of the enemy.

Now the soldier is, for all purposes, is AWOL [absent without leave] from his battalion in God's army. My extended study on Balu and my goal of working on gastro-esophageal reflux and hiatus hernia completely took God and His purpose off from my mind.

I justified that I was serving people and through them, God. I did not care to or ask if such was God's purpose for my life.

Laugh at Sin [the serpent]

Next, scene of the sin-show is to make the soldier to ridicule and **'laugh-at the sin show.'** The Devil wants one to laugh at sin instead of being repulsed. This 'pause' to laugh makes the soldier hesitate or stop. Pure revulsion will make one quickly leave that place.

The soldier who side steps from the marching column to pause looses time and his team. By now the troop has marched away, and the soldier is left, surrounded by people who have come to see the [sin] show.

These are actors in the show who are participant enemy soldiers and intend to trap the soldier.

I was not only involved deeply with the roadside performer; I had to document my findings. So I sought the help of the movie and film industry, making friends with a vast number of film producers, directors, script writers, music directors and of course numerous actors of both genders.

I am not calling all the above referred friends who helped me, loved and cared for me, even when I had no means of paying them adequately for their services, as sinners, or as enemies.

I am referring only about me, and my action of abandoning my commission given by God. God has eventually rectified matters. Just as these good friends had helped me, now I was enabled and burdened to pray with concern and care.

The next stage of T.V./Media trap was the show called 'Three is company'. The show starts with two young women and a man living together in one small apartment. It was an apparent comedy, but brought tragedy to many in the nation.

The show progressed to multiple partners living together a subtle diversion for people to accept multiple partners as an alternative to the marriage, which demands one man and one wife for the family.

This has become an alternate open home for a large number in many so called advanced countries. People live together as an alternative to marriage and its responsibility.

The next stage of T.V. viewing slid into watching the 'dating/ mating' games organized and run by pimps, offering big awards, wardrobes, and travel trips for the two unmarried people.

Laugh with Sin [the serpent]

The sin show is now changing gears to make the soldier '**laugh with, and get involved in the sin show**.' The soldier is overwhelmed by the enemy, made to become more attentive to the people around, and is beginning to tolerate, and even appreciate the bad jokes and comments that surround him.

The next step down the TV ladder, are 'talk shows' which generates wicked gossip and to wash many dirty linen in public. Glib talkers compete to bring abnormal male and female relationships into open shows, calling them cleverly as 'different points of view' to desensitize the public against morality.

Many soap operas have come into existence, to turn people's limited lifetime into crime time. In these shows, every one not in the house will be having affairs, out in the office or else where. The actors take over the minds of the watchers, to such an extent that the audience feels justified in cheating on their real mates who have gone out to work. This is one of the major causes of divorces and breakdown of homes.

Sin [Serpent] Laughs at You

The soldier by now is stranded as his troop has long been gone and he is at the mercy of Satan, hypnotized by the sinister Serpent. And **sin now laughs at** the soldier as he is taken captive and transported into the enemy concentration camp, surrounded by hordes of varying kinds of venomous serpents.

If you to the enemy serpent army surrender,
Surrounded you will be as the serpent's fodder.

When Satan shows you ways to win a match,
You be aware, that to him, 'you' are the catch.

This is followed by the present trend in TV's downhill shows where there are talks, and demands for freedom of speech and expression for every individual.

There are violent and virulent criticisms against the laws upholding or defending or maintaining fundamental morality by the same group demanding equal rights. Movies like 'deep throat' are considered as a form of classical art and not pornography, and even taken to the capital.

They are now making an intolerant out cry for liberation from morality. There are at the same breath aggressive demands for tolerance toward every kind of perversion and legalization for the rights of the perverts.

This gradual desensitization of morality has now resulted in promotion of pornography, protected and allowed even in public libraries for children. Our young children have become targets. Perverted [activist] judges have started legalizing infant sacrifices to the goddess [The lady of liberty,] to legitimize the freedom of choice for women who want pleasure, but not responsibility. Homosexuality is being accepted as alternate lifestyle, and enforced legally, and kindergarten children are inculcated to this trend with classes and videos. Families' homes and churches are dubbed as outdated entities in the modern scientific era.

Total self-centeredness is encouraged. Many games have developed and promoted openly to foster hatred that shapes the player into violence and murder, and, these are considered to be high-tech technology necessary for this century.

Sex has been reduced from a sacred responsibility to an elimination process and for instant gratification. Condoms are given like candies to the kids in some schools. Fundamental morality was been labeled as homophobic.

Those who want to live or consider moral life as an alternate life style are being dubbed as intolerant to hateful homophobic.

The final and seventh stage is to get rid of God and morality from the currency and the constitution. If these also become legal any one who feels like doing any thing has not broken any law, as there will be no law.

There would be no need to becoming a Christian. No need to have a war, if Christ is removed and Satan is made our ruler.

As I mentioned earlier, there are only two armies in the world. If you do not belong to God's army, you automatically and forcibly are drafted into the devil's army. One thing is for sure; there are no civilians.

So, by default, I was drawn into the enemy territory and made a captive and put to work by the enemy. Satan the eternal lethal serpent tightened his coils around me. To fatten me up, he set traps for me by opening up his alternatives in which I willingly indulged.

Very soon I realized that the enemy shackles and coils were getting tighter and tighter. I was put into chains and given no freedom of choice any more.

I remembered like the prodigal, the freedom of choice, which was given to me, when I was in the Father's home (God's army). This left me with depression and a sense of doom and damnation. I tried to read the Bible, but the sinister serpent, then came out to me with misinterpreted scriptures.

The serpent tried to convince me that there was no more hope for me to return to my previous association with God's army, and that I would be better off if I joined him and serve him.

The way he used me and wanted to use me was to sabotaging God's army and bring to him as many victims as captives as possible.

All the serpent wanted was to hurt the Leader of God's army in any way possible.

Gradually, I stopped reading the Bible, withdrew from worship, and started avoiding meeting with evangelical Christians. In any army, such a soldier is no more a prisoner of war, but a rank traitor deserving to face a firing squad.

As I was being sucked into this sewer, the good Lord reached out and restored me. More on this as we proceed.

My abandoned Leader did not press charges against me, but kept speaking-up for me. He was offering me a free pardon, if I returned. It is a tragedy that I did not return the love my Leader showed for me for many years. I was too embarrassed to repent and return. I took up a godless life style to justify existing even while I was in India.

I took-up sports and athletics to replace prayer and bible reading. I won the college individual championship at the Christian Medical College and later won the college blues of the Madras Medical College.

I was thinking of serious sports and athletics future when a motor vehicle accident and a broken spine made me understand that such was not to be my future. I was a poor student academically.

To my surprise I was invited to be on the faculty at the Christian Medical College in the radiology department.

What made it more surprising, unexpected and important to me was because it was the founder of the Christian Medical College, Dr. Ida S Scudder, who asked me to give few years of my life to help in the department of Radiology.

Dr, Donald Paterson, and Dr. Ida B. Scudder had build up the diagnostic and therapeutic sections against odds. So I did, knowing that it will be for more than few years. For, in those years Radiology was not a popular subject.

To be in academics it was necessary to get higher degrees. I was offered the Colombo-plan scholarship to do the British Radiology Faculty's fellowship training and pass the examination in London from the Royal College of Hammersmith Hospital.

On my return, I was made the chief of the radio-diagnostic section in the prestigious Christian Medical College Medical School and Hospital.

Dr. Patterson had retired by now, and I became busy in teaching, research and upgrading the department, and, making a name for my 'self'. I neglected God and my home, seeking academic honors.

This was the time I came across the roadside 'free serpent show' by Balu, and, that was my crutch, and excuse, till it broke.

BIG DREAM ON EARTH
BIG SCREAM IN DEATH

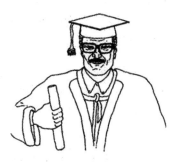

I have deliberately inserted some of the academic degrees I obtained - behind my name. It is not intended to tell others that I am a scholar, but that I have been only **a well-educated fool**, and a waster.

I spent most of my life; my time, my money and my efforts to get what can be called as academic "certificate of authenticity"! This was another flimsy crutch, and has no more use for me now.

I find to my great disappointment that the alphabets that represent **the degrees I collected so painfully and for so many years are 'behind me' in more then one sense, and have no more value to me, even when I am alive and active.**

In the five decades of academic medicine, I found that the questions had remained the same, where as there were final and definitive answers upheld by the highly acclaimed scholars, which changed at least once every decade.

The academicians are superbly nonchalant about the cutting edge of changing knowledge, making them into liars and fossils. Their bravado remains unruffled. Only con artists can maintain this arrogant put on such an attitude, not true scientists!

My medical textbooks are being revised every few months and even the recent, past information is trashed. I was really surprised that the Bible, which is more than 2000 years old, is still, current, needing no revision, or upgrading.

The teachings of the Bible are being hijacked, with no acknowledgement to the origin, and new "scientific" disciplines are started, to make the truths globally acceptable, for private profit and fame.

DON'T LOSE YOUR HEAD

Two great statesmen in Britain, and who were personal life long friends of kings were beheaded by their friendly kings. One a them had commented before loosing his head that if he had given half of the time to God which he gave the king, his head wouldn't have been parted from the body.

When to others in love you are attached
From your self-demand you are detached

We tend to, as I did **'loose our heads'** over sports, athletics, wealth, career, bank balances and academic achievements. None of these will matter, nor go with us into the future.

Anyone with wisdom, or even basic sense would and should be planning for the future, which should be really

the conclusion and inclusion of meaningful education, or, the acquirement of knowledge. This is the basis of understanding.

For 30 years I carried on, not caring whether the floods were one inch above my head, or one mile. I made my work my god, and, that, I understand now, is no substitute.

I was made an examiner in many universities in India and in other countries, I was invited to give lectures and participate in National and International conferences around the globe.

Popularity and position dragged me into an abyss of self-indulgence. I will not list or describe the depth of degradation the devil can take one into as he did me.

This book is not an advertisement for the devil the serpent. This writing is to emphasize that there is hope even for a notorious deserter and traitor.

And Heavenly prepared antivenin for even the most venomous bites of many spiritual serpents.

It is to expose some of the enemy serpent's strategies against the soldiers of God's army, and to show hope for the 'back-sliders'.

God has promised hope and pardon for any degree of sinner at any stage, who seeks His pardon.

When I thought that there was no more hope for me, as I was unable to walk or escape back to Him, from the bottom of hell where I was kept a captive, the Lord Jesus, and the Holy Spirit came, breaking through all barriers and rescued me.

They carried me out as I was not even strong enough to crawl, leave alone walk back to my old barracks in God's army.

If you trust in God
Then you rest in God

The enemy serpent, the accuser and the devil, filed charges against me, that according to the military law, I should be court-martialed and executed, or, turned over to him. He quoted the universal scriptural-law of "corrupted graft of wine has to be burned down!"

ROASTED ON THE FIRE

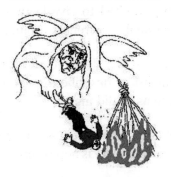

It is a fact that the branch (me) that God grafted into Himself (the Tree) bore bad fruits, and also bore poisonous fruits. Rightly so, Satan the serpent demanded that the army rules be followed (for my desertion and betrayal) and that the corrupted branch be cut down and burnt in 'his hell' quoting the Scriptural law put in the Bible, [for his pound of flesh].

When for wrong things you get a burning desire,
You are getting setup, to be cast into eternal fire.

As a result, I suffered three massive heart attacks with death of some parts of the heart muscles, which, even surgery could not correct. But even as the devil was dancing around me in the flames of hell, God pulled me out, an almost burnt-out branch, a charred dirty piece of charcoal, to use as a chalk to pen His message of hope and His never changing love and promises to those who have trusted Him.

Satan the serpent presumed that he plucked me off from God's hand! But that is not possible. For, I am a witness and an example to God's unfathomable power and immense grace.

Miscalculations of Mesmerizing Serpent the Mammon.

God, He lovingly grafted me to the eternal Vine
When through grace He entered this heart of mine
He called me 'son' through His love Divine
And delighted as the graft's tendrils with the Vine twine.

Rom.11: 17

But the graft went sour, and sour grapes on it hung
So, it had to be properly pruned and cut
The trimmed off branches into flames were flung
Satan rejoiced that from God's hands me he plucked out.

Rom.11: 20-22.

The Master, the Maker, from the ashes He took,
The charred branch, and to His purpose made use,
As He on His canvas, for all to take a look
Did outline the fact that His love is too profuse,
To cast-out any who in their lives, God did choose.

Rom.11: 23

Again the Devil, on his plans to cut God to his own puny size,
Found that he cannot ever God's plans fathom-out ,
Nor pluck-out a wandering sheep of God as his own prize,
Nor can he at any time, against God, win or luck-out.

Rom.11: 29.

Zec.3:2-4. "And the Lord said to Satan, "I, the Lord, reject your accusations, Satan. Yes, the Lord, who has chosen Jerusalem, rebukes you. This man is like a burning stick that has been snatched from afire."

Because of my spiritual wounds and scars, which have crippled me, God has given me now a secretarial post. I am afraid, I write too slowly and make a lot of spelling mistakes and incomplete sentences, but He is very patient and kind and puts up with me! What a Master to serve!

The clerical job given to me is to:

(1) Write out His message, on a board using even me, the burnt-out, still a dirty piece of coal used as a chalk, to other victims and even active soldiers.

(2) Cross-out [at the Cross], Shade-out (blot-out the wrong notions leading to of lose of hope of other similar AWOLS - (absent without leave) backsliders, and to let them know that there is hope for all, in all situations, however bad it may be.

(3) To give warning about the pending 'fire-treatment' to other corrupt branches using me the "still smoking branch, plucked out of hell" as a torch. (God even uses utterly hopeless subjects like myself.)

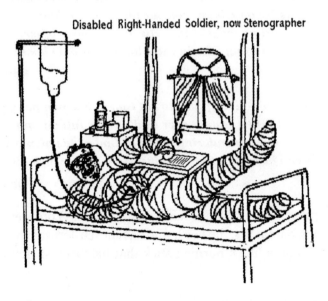

Disabled Right-Handed Soldier, now Stenographer

So, for no other earthly reason, but because of heavenly grace and mercy beyond human or the serpent-devil's understanding, God pulled me out of, not only an untimely death, but out of the uttermost bottom of hell, so that I can tell others that even in such sin-sink-holes, that **"to God, there is no hopeless situation"**.

In the Old Testament, we see that Moses was ordered to lift up the brass serpent in the desert to the dying Israelites so that they could live.

The people were not called to worship the serpents, or to put their hope on a man made snake-idols or icons.

They were to see and acknowledge their reason for dying, was that they were being bitten to death is by the **serpent's bite called 'Sin.'**

To avoid death, they had **to confess their sins** (grumbling, ingratitude, seeking the idols of Egypt, and flesh pots etc.) and **to repent**, in order to be healed, and to survive.

I am sharing this message [of healing from the serpent-bite more than once and having survived] with others, to hear, heed, and see their own need.

All I can say to you is "Don't look at the messenger [me], but look at the one who has sent you this message, for your healing and eternal life".

Why Not End Your Own Hopelessness
For, In God, You Do Have Hope, Endless.

ACCUSED IS EXCUSED

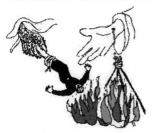

MY SAVIOR'S SACRED BLOOD DID FLOW TO DRENCH ALL THE HELL'S FIRES, AROUND ME, TO DRENCH

When you, my reader, really commit your life to God, repent of your sin, confess them, and ask Him to come into your heart and life, He will do so **even though He knows how unsteady you may be in the future.**

Your job right now is to invite Him into your heart, **not only as a Resident, but also as the all-powerful President.**

Then, God takes it upon Himself, as His job, to protect you and provide for you. The serpent may use your pride, selfishness etc. to bite, or shoot you in your foot to keep you from marching in God's army, giving you plenty of lame excuses to waste your valuable, irreplaceable time.

When the serpent finds that he cannot steal your eternal life from God's hand, he will try his best to steal the time, which God has given to you on this earth to serve Him and fulfill the purpose for which you had been created. (The serpent brought death into the world, and therefore he can steal your time on earth from you).

The devil will try to deliver death to your time when he finds that you escaped eternal death by receiving the Lord Jesus into your heart. One needs to fear death of time more than ones' inevitable mortal death from this world.

The devil steals our prime time To use it as his crime-time

Yes, the serpent bit the '**sole**' of my foot and convinced me that he got my '**soul**' (for nearly 40 years). I had been telling myself it was too late, and that my recurrent sin was, too great.

The serpent would not allow me to think any further, escalating my megalomaniac attitude, making me believe that '**MY**' sins were too much, **even for God** to understand and forgive.

This thinking I now realize is not due to humility or to any thing laudable, but due to an arrogant and subtle pride that makes me feel that, good or bad, I am still the greatest, even above God the Maker and the Creator.

*If your spiritual life is ailing
It is because your faith is failing.*

The serpent knows that God does not approve of pride and therefore goads everyone on, to invite various forms of pride into their thoughts, words and actions.

The serpent's bites to make me to double-cross God, brought, me to [double-back to] the real Cross again, and by sheer grace, mercy, and His faithfulness', God reopened my eyes to see truth and to acknowledge my proper priorities.

Now, when God brings in situations where He wants to use me to help others by pointing them to God with my words or acts, or, pass-on to them His message, I still catch myself giving lame excuses that "I am not worthy etc."

The Lord gently reminds me "a soldier is only expected to obey and not expected to analyze or offer alternate solutions". The healths of my soul or, the other excuses I may cook-up, are equivalent to insubordination in the battlefield situation.

We need to remember in our daily prayer that we live our daily life in the battlefield of spiritual warfare.

*When Satan shows you ways to win a match \
You be aware that to him, 'you' are the catch*

I once in desperation cried "God please listen only to my cry; please don't look at who is crying, and where I am crying from" Now, I realize it was only the echo from heaven, and God didn't want me to see me through my own wretched self; for He hears and looks at me and others like me only through the One, by whom we were enlisted, the Lord Jesus, God's son, and my Leader, who rescued me and vouches for me eternally.

He is the One who enlisted me as well as others like me. He gave His life for me, still loves me, and is not ready to abandon me to the enemy, however far the distance the enemy may have kidnapped and taken me.

The army recruitment slogan says, "Be all you can be". But this is possible only if one is in God's army.

What more can I say? Yes, **'the pension benefits are just out of this world and extended for ever into eternity!'**

There is no fear of bankruptcy of 'social security, or prohibitive health costs. There is free board and lodge. Neither the serpent, nor his army will be there to harm any one. What better plans for your present and future can you think of? The answer of course is none. So Join God's army – today, right now.

When to God you are fully yielded
From Satan, you are fully shielded

To escape the serpent, to Join God's army, or be reinstated; sincerely pray the following prayer:

"Dear God, our Father, my sins have dragged me far away from You, and made me become Your enemy.

I have hurt and grieved You by my numerous and repeated sins.

I repent and confess all my sins, and for being a deserter and a betrayer.

I know that nothing is hid from your sight.

I make no excuses.

Please forgive me and make me a new creature in You.

I desire to return Your love and serve You faithfully with all of my heart.

Help me to take You Lord Jesus as the owner of my life and enable me to follow You.

Thank You for dying on the Cross for me.

Thank You for rising again from death for me, on earth itself, to hear my prayer.

I pray this prayer from my repentant heart.

Make my heart become the humble abode for You and the Holy-Spirit.

Please accept me as I come seeking Thy mercy and I come "Just as I am without one plea or excuse".

In Jesus Christ's name I pray. Amen.

Even an end can become a start
When prayer comes from the heart

This is the true-life story of the author. If you need to write to the author he will be more than happy to help you in your decision to live for the Lord Jesus. This may not be possible for many of the readers. I would like to make the following recommendations:

- Find a church that believes in the Bible, in the saving grace of the Lord Jesus Christ, and become an active member.

- Join or form a small prayer group and have regular prayers, if possible on a daily basis.

- Read the Bible daily. I find it a blessing to read it while I'm on my knees.

- Give your witness as to how God forgave and saved you. Share it with people on every occasion.

- Build a firewall [prayer wall] around you and your near and dear ones.

- Remember you are a copper wire. Only when you are in contact with the power line [God], power will flow through you to others.

Email: johnops5l@yahoo.com
Website: http://www.healingfacts.org
        http://www.healingfacts.com

– **A.C. JOHNSON,** M.D., Ph.D., F. F. R.

ACKNOWLEDGEMENT

My thanks are due to

- Pastor John Paul, International Ministries.

- Mr. Leslie Samuel, my co-worker in the service of our Lord, who proof reads, formats, works with graphics, and web design.

- Dr. Satyabama Johnson. FRCP, my patient, long-suffering wife.

- Professor G. V. Rajendran Thirunelveli – India.

- Dr. Wad of Haffkine Institute – Bombay, India.

- Mr. Romulus Whitaker – Snake farm, Chennai, India.

- Professor P. J. Deoras – Haffkine Institute, Bombay, India.

- Mr. Durai Pandithurai, Assistant Financial Secretary, DHQ, TX, USA, Salvation Army.

- The family and friends who provided for and supported me;

- The artist, Mr. Paneerselvam. – Chennai, India.

- Mr. Dhoondi & Mr. Sunderlal Nahata, Cine Film Producers and their team.

- The technical, paramedical, and medical staff of the Radiology Department of the Christian Medical College & Hospital, Vellore, India.

- The circus & the roadside performers – India.

- The many children of God who faithfully bring to us God's messages.

If I have to acknowledge all those used by God to help me write this book, I will need another large volume. I will reserve my thanks to be conveyed, personally – when we meet in heaven.